TOP KNIFE

THE ART & CRAFT OF TRAUMA SURGERY

Asher Hirshberg MD

&

Kenneth L. Mattox MD

Edited by Mary K. Allen

Illustrated by Scott Weldon

tfm Publishing Ltd, Castle Hill Barns, Harley, Nr Shrewsbury, SY5 6LX, UK.
Tel: +44 (0)1952 510061; Fax: +44 (0)1952 510192
E-mail: nikki@tfmpublishing.com; Web site: www.tfmpublishing.com

Editor:	Mary K Allen
Design and layout:	Nikki Bramhill
Cover design:	Scott Weldon

Illustrations by Scott Weldon, Copyright © Baylor College of Medicine 2005

Paperback	ISBN-10:	1-903378-22-2
	ISBN-13:	978-1-903378-22-9

E-book editions: 2015		
ePub	ISBN:	978-1-903378-90-8
Mobi	ISBN:	978-1-903378-91-5
Web pdf	ISBN:	978-1-903378-92-2

NOTICE

Neither the authors, nor the publisher, nor any other party who has been involved in the preparation or publication of this work can accept responsibility for any injury or damage to persons or property occasioned through the implementation of any ideas or use of any product described herein. Neither can they accept any responsibility for errors, omissions or misrepresentations, howsoever caused.

Whilst every care is taken by the authors, the editors and the publisher to ensure that all information and data in this book are as accurate as possible at the time of going to press, it is recommended that readers seek independent verification of advice on drug or other product usage, surgical techniques and clinical processes prior to their use.

Contents

Contributors

Authors

Asher Hirshberg MD FACS, is Professor in the Department of Surgery, SUNY Downstate College of Medicine and Director of Emergency Vascular Surgery at Kings County Hospital Center in Brooklyn, New York.

Kenneth L. Mattox MD FACS, is Professor and Vice Chair of the Michael E. DeBakey Department of Surgery, Baylor College of Medicine, and Chief of Staff/Chief of Surgery at the Ben Taub General Hospital, Houston, Texas.

Illustrator

Scott Weldon MA, is Supervisor Medical Illustrator in the Division of Cardiothoracic Surgery of the Michael E. DeBakey Department of Surgery, Baylor College of Medicine, Houston, Texas.

Editor

Mary K. Allen BA, is Administrative Associate in the Michael E. DeBakey Department of Surgery, Baylor College of Medicine, and Administrator of the Surgery Division at the Ben Taub General Hospital, Houston, Texas.

To our residents -

past, present and future

Introduction

What this Book is all About

When you have to shoot - shoot, don't talk

~ Eli Wallach (Tuco)
in: *The Good, the Bad and the Ugly,* 1966

Sooner or later, it happens.

You are a young attending surgeon doing your first night on call at a busy trauma center or a surgeon in a community hospital facing a bad trauma case alone and without backup. Perhaps you are a military surgeon with a Forward or Field Surgical Team. Sooner or later, you find yourself in the operating room (OR) with a massively bleeding patient rapidly dying in your hands.

You quickly open the belly and blood gushes out. Loops of bowel are swimming in a pool of dark blood and clots. Hectic activity surrounds you as the anesthesiology team struggles to open more lines while the operating room nurses rapidly deploy instrument trays. You don't need to look at the alarming numbers on the monitor to realize that this is *The Moment*. The skills that you have worked so hard to acquire are suddenly put to a very brutal test. Can you meet the challenge?

These cases almost invariably roll through the emergency room (ER) doors when you feel you are not at your best. You are tired and running on auxiliary batteries. Your scrub nurse is "not very experienced." The anesthesiologists are doing their best by pushing bolus after bolus of a particularly nasty inotropic agent. The circulating nurse disappeared off the radar screen five minutes ago in search of your favorite vascular clamp. Yes, this is definitely not a good time, but we can assure you, it never is. The audible bleeding in the belly, the controlled chaos around you, the blinking red lights in your head, and the clueless assistant across the operating table are all part of real-life trauma surgery. Oh, and by the way, have you noticed the anorexic chap in the black robe and hood, standing in the corner of the OR, holding this big scythe, and patiently waiting for you to make just one mistake? He, too, is an integral part of trauma surgery.

Trauma surgery is an art that combines decision-making with technical and leadership skills. The purpose of this book is to help you take a badly wounded patient to the OR, organize yourself and your team, do battle with some vicious injuries, and come out with a live patient and the best possible result. The standard surgical atlas may show you what to do with your hands but not how to think, plan, and improvise. This book is different. Here you will find practical advice on how to use your head as well as your hands when you are operating on a crashing trauma patient.

Who should read this book? Are you a resident or registrar in the senior years of surgical training? A general surgeon interested in trauma? A fellow in trauma and critical care? If you are, we wrote this book primarily with you in mind.

If you are currently in training, you must be aware of the strong forces dramatically reducing your operative trauma experience. Urban penetrating trauma is declining, non-operative management is on the rise, and surgical training is undergoing a noisy revolution. While this book cannot substitute for getting your clogs wet in a real OR, it can optimize the educational value of every trauma operation you do because you will come prepared.

Many operative encounters with bad injuries take place in austere circumstances. The rural surgeon doing an occasional major trauma case alone, the military surgeon in the field, and the disaster relief team on a humanitarian mission are examples of trauma surgery with extremely limited resources. Tackling a high-grade liver injury in a large trauma center is bad enough. Doing it in the only OR of a 20-bed hospital takes tons of courage and resourcefulness. If you are one of those surgeons, you are probably more interested in simple technical solutions that work, rather than complex maneuvers that you won't use anyway. Most operative problems in trauma have more than one effective answer, and the trick is to tailor a simple, feasible solution to your specific circumstances. In this book, we show you how to do just that.

This brings us to damage control, the biggest buzzword in trauma surgery in the last decade. You may wonder why you don't see a chapter on damage control in the book. The answer is simple. Damage control has become such a central theme in trauma surgery that it no longer makes sense to confine it to a single chapter. Instead, detailed descriptions of damage control options and techniques are part of every chapter. Thinking of this book as a comprehensive guide to damage control would not be a mistake.

Why *Top Knife*? Top Gun is the popular name of the Naval Fighters Weapons School. Their mission is to train the very best fighter pilots for the US Navy. We called our book *Top Knife* in recognition of the many similarities between trauma surgeons and fighter pilots: clear thinking under pressure, responding effectively to rapidly changing situations, and a long and arduous training process. Just like aerial combat, trauma surgery is, first and foremost, a discipline. You cannot become a fighter pilot or trauma surgeon without a lot of hard work and willingness to face adversity.

The book begins and ends in the OR. If you are looking for information on care of the injured patient before or after the operation, look elsewhere. We also assume that you are familiar with general surgical principles and techniques. If you seek instruction on how to resect and join bowel or how to do a standard vascular anastomosis, you will not find it here. However, if you wish to learn how to do a no-nonsense crash laparotomy, deal with a bleeding lung, or repair an injured popliteal artery, read on.

The first section of the book, *Tools of the Trade*, presents principles of trauma surgery that cut across injury types and anatomical areas. Our focus is not so much on how you should be sewing, but rather on how you should be thinking and reacting. These skills are rarely if ever taught in surgical training. If anyone ever showed you how to develop an alternative plan while struggling with a bleeding subclavian artery or to pay attention to what the circulating nurse is doing while you are manually compressing a shattered liver, consider yourself very fortunate. Most surgical residents and registrars are expected to just intuitively pick up those skills somewhere along the way. Many never do.

The rest of the book is about trauma surgery as a contact sport. Here we show you how to deal with specific injuries. An important theme is how things can go wrong, an aspect of trauma surgery seldom addressed in standard texts. We emphasize pitfalls because recognizing them is an essential part of learning to operate.

We acknowledge that the art and craft of trauma surgery vary among surgeons. Don't be surprised to find some differences in the approaches to operative problems between the authors. The underlying principles are the same, but techniques are sometimes different. Where such variations exist, we have pointed them out. No one size fits all.

In developing this book we had the good fortune to partner with Scott Weldon, an extraordinarily gifted young medical illustrator. The translation of surgical ideas and concepts into graphical form is always a tricky business. Thanks to Scott's talent and superb intuition, we were able to express this author-artist partnership as a single voice that seamlessly interweaves text and art.

Mary Allen, the most talented editor we have ever worked with, did some radical surgery on the text and mercilessly beat it into shape until she got it just right. Without her remarkable efforts, this book would have been much longer - and considerably less readable.

Nikki Bramhill, our publisher, was a full participant in this project from the embryonic stages to the final product. She bought into our idea to write an informal "eye level" operative book on trauma surgery and worked with us every step of the way to make it happen. Her infectious enthusiasm, hard work, and superb eye are evident on every page.

And now, it's time to stop talking - and start cutting ...

Chapter 1

The 3-D Trauma Surgeon

An expert is a man who has made all possible mistakes in a very narrow field.

-- Neils Bohr

The first thing you notice on entering the peritoneal cavity is bleeding from a large nasty hole in the right lobe of the liver. Strangely enough, you were in exactly the same situation a week ago. You don't even have to glance at the monitor to know the systolic pressure is going to be 60. Remembering last week's case, you rapidly pack the liver to stop the bleeding. However, this time the injured liver continues to bleed through the packs. It was supposed to stop. It did last week. What's wrong? What's different? You do a Pringle maneuver, but it doesn't help much. The metallic voice of the anesthesiologist alerts you that the patient's systolic pressure is now unobtainable. He is dying. What is going on? What do you do now?

You remain surprisingly calm for a surgical resident with only three or four years of training. The reason is simple: you know exactly what comes next. Soon the lights in the Surgical Virtual Reality Lab will be turned on and the simulation will pause. Using a revolving hologram of the injured liver and retrohepatic veins, your instructor will explain what went wrong and why. This "dry clogs" approach to teaching surgery is rapidly becoming a major part of surgical training. A simulator can help you learn to operate, yet something fundamental is missing.

When you work on a simulator, operate in a large animal lab, or work in the OR with a good teaching assistant, you learn the tactical dimension of the operation. You learn to select from several technical options and execute your choice in specific operative circumstances. You spend most of your surgical training focused on operative tactics in elective and emergency procedures. Only when you begin operating on your own do you become aware of the other two dimensions of every operation: strategy and team leadership.

The strategic dimension of an operation is the broad consideration of goals, means, and alternatives. When you operate with a teaching assistant, your teacher usually handles the strategic dimension for you. While you are absorbed in mobilizing the splenic flexure, your teacher is already weighing the options of a rapid damage control laparotomy against a time-consuming definitive repair.

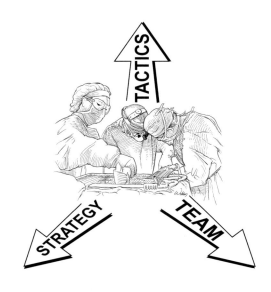

When you are working on your own, the strategic dimension suddenly falls on your shoulders. You can no longer focus exclusively on the holes in the colon, but must also consider the "Big Picture."

The third dimension of every operation is team leadership. Being a surgeon means making sure that the efforts of the OR team members are coordinated and focused on the same goals. You cannot assume your scrub tech knows what to do next just because he or she is smart and experienced. You must clearly communicate your plan. Similarly, the anesthesiologist does not have extrasensory perception and cannot guess your plan unless you share it. Mishandling the team dimension during a trauma operation is one of the worst mistakes you can make.

To operate effectively on wounded patients, you must train yourself to be a 3-dimensional surgeon who constantly zooms in and out of the tactical, strategic, and team dimensions, monitoring progress and reassessing options in each.

Putting brain in gear before knife in motion

Strategic thinking is essential even before you make the incision. Consider, for example, the "black hole" of surgery, a term you have never heard yet encounter every day. The black hole is the time between the patient's entry into the OR and the skin incision. It is an obligatory logistic interval during which the patient is moved, positioned, and prepared, but nothing is done to stop internal bleeding

If you choose to spend most of the black hole interval at the scrub sink, you may end up with clean fingernails, but when you enter the OR you will find the patient improperly positioned, the scrub nurse prepping the wrong field, and the OR team effort in disarray. You may well have lost the battle before firing your first shot. To avoid this, stay with your patient until the last possible moment and use the black hole for effective preparations.

Is the patient positioned properly? Does the OR team know which operative field to prepare and which instrument sets to deploy? Does the anesthesia team need help with lines? You cannot address these questions from the scrub sink. Go and scrub only when you are sure that everything is set up and ready.

If the patient is in shock, don't waste time on scrubbing. Every second counts. Just get a gown and gloves, grab a knife, and rapidly dive into the chest or abdomen.

Sterility is a luxury in severe hemorrhagic shock

The way you position the patient and define the operative field are other indicators of your strategic vision. Always prepare for a worst-case scenario. In torso trauma, this typically involves access to both sides of the diaphragm and to the groins. Your worst-case operative field extends from the chin to above the knees,

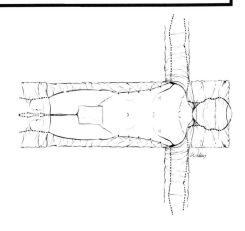

between the posterior axillary lines. Abduct both arms to allow the anesthesiology team full access to the upper extremities.

For isolated extremity trauma, include the entire injured extremity in the field to facilitate manipulation, and prepare an uninjured lower extremity for saphenous vein harvesting. For a neck exploration, prepare the entire chest, since the upper mediastinum is a continuation of the neck.

Always prep for a worst-case scenario

ABC of tactical thinking

Train yourself to think of every operation as a sequence of well-defined steps, but memorizing the steps is not enough. You must gain insight into the procedure by learning the key maneuver and the pitfall in every step.

A *key maneuver* is the single most important technical act in an operative step. The key maneuver in mobilizing an injured spleen is incising the splenorenal ligament and entering the correct plane between the spleen and the kidney. Often, a key maneuver is identifying a gatekeeper, a structure that serves as a guide to dissection or opens the correct tissue plane. The gatekeeper of the carotid artery in the neck is the common facial vein. Identifying and dividing it is the key maneuver. When mobilizing the hepatic flexure of the colon, the key maneuver is finding the plane between the right side of the transverse colon and the duodenum.

A *pitfall* is a major trap that awaits you in every operative step. Choosing an incorrect thoracotomy incision or performing it at the wrong intercostal space is a major pitfall. Failure to obtain proximal control before plunging into a contained hematoma is another classic trap.

Familiarity with both the key maneuver and classic pitfall of every operative step is the difference between the trauma pro and the wannabe. Knowing the key maneuvers and pitfalls of a procedure allows you to perform the procedure independently and, with experience, teach it to others.

Know the key maneuver and pitfall in every operative step

A common tactical dilemma

Have you ever heard of flailing? Flailing is repetitive, ineffective action. It is one of the most common tactical errors of the inexperienced. For example, imagine yourself trying to control a bleeder with a hemostatic stitch. You insert the suture and tie it, but bleeding continues. You try again. It still doesn't work. You try again; maybe it will work this time. We can tell you without being there that it probably won't - you are flailing. Very often, flailing will be more obvious to the OR team than to you. How can you avoid it?

Get used to the idea that in the real world surgical maneuvers don't always work. Even the most technically gifted surgeon does not succeed in every move. You must learn to deal with technical failure effectively, not emotionally. When a maneuver doesn't work, don't take it as a personal failure. Pause and consider your options.

First, reconsider the need for the failed act. Is it really necessary? Does the bleeder require a suture? Perhaps it will stop with temporary pressure and patience.

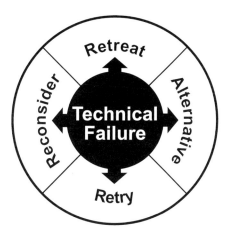

Another option is to retreat and get help. If you are fortunate enough to have backup, use it. Someone more experienced often has a better chance of solving the problem. Recognizing the need for help and asking for it (whether you are a resident or seasoned trauma surgeon), is a sign of good judgment.

What if you are completely on your own and help is not an option? Then you must consider alternative techniques or a different approach to the problem. If your original solution doesn't work, you must come up with one that will.

How about trying again? As a rule, repeating an act or maneuver that has failed is worthwhile only if you have changed something in the tactical environment: better exposure, an improved angle, a longer needle driver, a bigger needle, or a better assistant. Such a tactical change improves your chance to succeed in the next attempt. Identical repetition of an unsuccessful technical act is a mistake because it almost always fails. This is the very definition of flailing and exactly what you must avoid.

Remember these four options for dealing with technical failure. They are your tickets out of frustrating and dangerous situations. Effective surgeons don't take technical failure as a personal insult. They rapidly reassess the situation and come up with an alternative solution.

Avoid flailing; learn to deal with technical failure

Tactical flexibility

Regardless of your experience, you will find yourself in situations where your inventory of standard techniques simply will not solve the problem, forcing you to figure out a new solution. Tactical flexibility is the ability to devise new solutions to unusual operative situations. It is an acquired skill that you can develop by learning to think outside the box.

When facing an unfamiliar problem, ask yourself the following questions:

◆ Have I encountered a similar situation in another context? In elective surgery? In another injured organ or anatomical region?
◆ Can I modify or adapt a standard technique to the situation?
◆ How about solving part of the problem?
◆ Can I leave the problem unsolved for a while and come back later?
◆ What is the minimal acceptable option to deal with the problem? Will draining the injury (and creating a controlled fistula) be good enough? Can I ligate the vessel instead of repairing it?

In a complex situation, always strive to simplify the problem. Assess the injuries and decide which injured organs must be fixed and which can be rapidly removed (or resected) and, thus, eliminated from the equation.

Make your reconstructions as simple as possible. The fewer suture lines you make, the better. In trauma surgery, simple solutions work; complex solutions often backfire on you.

Simplify complex tactical situations

The key strategic decision

Every trauma operation follows a generic sequence of reproducible steps. You gain access to the injured cavity, control bleeding and spillage using temporary measures, and then explore the cavity to define the injuries.

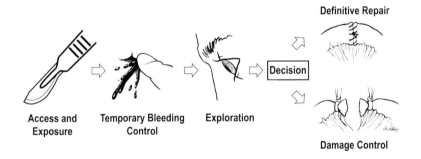

Now you face the key strategic decision of the operation, the choice between definitive repair and damage control. *Definitive repair* means resection or repair of the injured organs and formal closure of the cavity. *Damage control* means rapid bail out using temporary control measures and temporary closure of the cavity, with a planned return later under more favorable circumstances. You must make this decision very early. Don't find yourself abruptly bailing out in mid-operation because the patient is crashing.

How do you choose the operative profile? Consider four key factors: injury pattern, trauma burden, physiology, and system.

◆ What is the injury pattern?
For example, in a high-grade liver injury, once you recognize the need

for packing, damage control is your only choice. Similarly, the combination of a major abdominal vascular injury and intestinal perforations usually requires a rapid bail out, because by the time you finish dealing with the injured iliac artery, the patient will be in no condition to undergo bowel resection and anastomosis.

◆ What is the patient's overall trauma burden?

Look into the injured belly: how many organs do you need to fix? How much work is involved? What about the chest? Any pressing concerns in the limbs? The patient may need two hours of reconstructive work, but with a head injury and a dilated right pupil, you don't have the time. The overall trauma burden of a patient is a combination of the injuries, their relative urgency, and the amount of work (and time) required to deal with them. Investing precious time in definitive repair of non-life threatening abdominal injuries in the presence of big uncertainties in the head, chest, or neck is a very bad move.

◆ What is the patient's physiology?

The numbers you see on the anesthesiologist's monitor are not very helpful because you are not interested in a snapshot of the patient's blood pressure or oxygen saturation. You are interested in the physiological impact of the injury over time. The instantaneous numbers you see on the monitor mean very little. More on this in the next section.

◆ What system and circumstances are in play?

Are you an experienced trauma surgeon working in a trauma center or a general surgeon operating in a tent in Africa? How much blood do you have? How good is your anesthesiologist? You must incorporate these considerations into your decision. Damage control is the "great equalizer" of trauma surgery, allowing you to compensate for inexperience and limited resources.

> **Damage control is the great equalizer of trauma surgery**

The decision to bail out and the physiological envelope

If the patient's current blood pressure is 120/70 with good oxygen saturation, the anesthesiologist will often tell you the patient is stable. What if this patient was in shock for an hour before the operation and lost an entire blood volume before you gained control? Are you going to do a bowel resection and anastomosis? If you answer, "Yes," please say you are joking. This seemingly "stable" patient has, in fact, sustained a terrible physiological blow, and the systemic inflammatory response is going to hit full blast very soon. The bowel and the abdominal wall will swell, oxygenation will drop, and the patient will require massive fluid resuscitation and perhaps even inotropic support. You have to bail out and get the patient to the intensive care unit NOW! Your assessment of the cumulative physiological insult, not the numbers on the monitor screen, should guide your decision.

In the damage control literature there is much discussion of the "lethal triad" of hypothermia, coagulopathy, and acidosis. These three physiological derangements mark the boundaries of the patient's physiological envelope, beyond which there is irreversible shock and death. A core temperature below 32°C during a trauma laparotomy is considered universally fatal. Unfortunately, in real-life

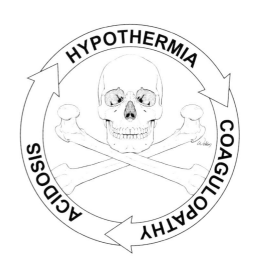

trauma surgery the lethal triad does not help you much. If you have a sound strategic grasp of the situation, you will bail out well before the patient's physiological envelope is anywhere near the point of no return. Being forced out of the chest by a core temperature of 33°C, a pH of 6.9, and a desperate anesthesiologist is not a sign of good judgment. You should have been out of that chest long ago.

Don't use the lethal triad as a guide to bailing out

Instead of the lethal triad, rely on a series of subtle perceptual cues to indicate a developing hostile physiology.

Intraoperative Cues of Hostile Physiology

Edema of the bowel mucosa
Midgut distension
Dusky serosal surfaces
Tissues cold to the touch
Non-compliant swollen abdominal wall
Diffuse oozing from surgical incisions

Edema and distension of the small bowel are relatively early warning signs, whereas diffuse oozing from the operative incision is a late one.

Experienced trauma surgeons decide on damage control within minutes of entering the abdomen and sometimes even before making the incision! They often recognize a pattern of injury and physiology that, in their experience, almost always leads to damage control. More on this in the chapter on thoracoabdominal injuries.

How well does your solution fail?

If you choose an operative profile of definitive repair, there is usually more than one repair option. The typical dilemma is between a shorter, simpler repair and a complex and more time-consuming reconstruction.

When choosing between several technical solutions, consider not only how well a particular option works but, more importantly, how well it *fails*. What will happen if the anastomosis leaks? What if the repaired spleen begins to bleed again?

There is a world of difference between a leaking colonic suture line and a failed pancreaticojejunostomy. The former is easily salvaged by proximal diversion; the latter is a much more ominous complication, not easy to manage. Can your patient tolerate a failure? A young healthy patient with an isolated bowel injury will survive a leak from a gastrointestinal (GI) suture line. A critically injured patient in multi-organ failure will not.

> **Choose a definitive repair option that fails well**

Team leadership

Picture yourself going head-to-head with an inaccessible hole in an iliac vein deep down in the pelvis. Your patient is in profound shock and bleeding audibly. Your team has one circulating nurse. Depending on your next request, the nurse will either go hunting for your personalized needle driver that has the ideal angle for your next 2-3 bites, bring a Fogarty balloon catheter that can free your finger from compressing the bleeder, or hook up an autotransfusion device. Which is more important? One circulator, three essential pieces of equipment needed at the same time - it's your call.

Constantly re-evaluate your priorities and your team, adapt to the situation, and make compromises. It is often said that excellent surgeons "can operate with a knife and fork." Is the special clamp you requested really essential? Can you get by with a less optimal but immediately available clamp? What will you need in five minutes? In ten minutes?

The key to a smooth and well-coordinated operation is to stay ahead of the game. As a rule, the scrub nurse should be at least one step ahead of the operation at any given moment. When you are exposing an injured vessel, the scrub nurse must already have clamps for proximal and distal control. The circulating nurse must be at least two steps ahead, making sure that the Fogarty balloon catheter and the sutures you will need for thrombectomy and repair are ready. You, the surgeon, must be at least three steps ahead, considering your reconstructive options. Just as in chess, the better player you are, the further ahead of the operation you will stay.

> **Stay well ahead of the operation**

Maintain a continuous dialogue with the anesthesiology team across the drape they call "the blood-brain barrier," and provide them with the information they need to stay ahead of the operation. Remember that you are working in one of several potentially injured cavities, and often the only clue that something is amiss in another visceral compartment will be obvious only to the anesthesiologist. Train yourself to listen to the monitor while you are working and to pick up any unusual moves or noises on the other side of the blood-brain barrier. Sometimes the most critical part of the operation is taking place there, outside your field of vision. While you cannot see it, you can train yourself to *feel* it.

Frequent changes in the operative plan are a salient feature of surgery for trauma, and it is your responsibility to make sure that members of the OR team are not left behind when the operative plan suddenly changes. Avoid surprises by sharing your tactical and strategic decisions with them. Consider, for example, the simple act of transporting a damage control patient to the surgical intensive care unit (SICU). If the team is unaware of your intention to bail out well in advance, you will find yourself in the ridiculous situation of having just performed a lightening-speed damage control laparotomy, only to spend an almost equal amount of time waiting for a bed.

Unlike chess, trauma surgery is a dynamic process. In chess, the pieces are just sitting there, waiting for you to make a move. A trauma operation moves forward relentlessly whether you like it or not, confronting you with rapidly changing situations. If you are an effective 3-D surgeon, your handling of the tactical, strategic, and teamwork dimensions translates into a smooth and effective procedure.

THE KEY POINTS

▶   Sterility is a luxury in severe hemorrhagic shock.

▶   Always prep for a worst-case scenario.

▶   Know the key maneuver and pitfall in every operative step.

▶   Avoid flailing; learn to deal with technical failure.

▶   Simplify complex tactical situations.

▶   Damage control is the "great equalizer" of trauma surgery.

▶   Don't use the "lethal triad" as a guide to bailing out.

▶   Choose a definitive repair option that fails well.

▶   Stay well ahead of the operation.

Chapter 2

Stop That Bleeding!

Whenever you encounter massive bleeding, the first thing to remember is: it's not your blood.

~ Raphael Adar, MD, FACS

In 1989, while discussing a paper on liver injuries, Dr. Francis Carter Nance of New Orleans made the following comment:

"I would like to offer Nance's classification of injuries, which has the advantage of not needing to look at the organ injured, but at the resident who is there at the operating table... If he or she looks at the wound and yawns and turns it over to the junior resident, then…it is going to do well. It is going to have a high survival rate. If he looks at the injury and salivates…that means that the resident will have to do some suturing and really help the patient, and the mortality rate will not be high, and he or she will look good during the morbidity-mortality conference. If the resident sweats…that means that he or she will do a lot of sewing, will encounter a complication, and will have to defend himself or herself at the morbidity-mortality conference, and probably receive a lot of heat. And if the resident screams and asks for the attending…you know that the patient will do poorly."

(*Ann Surg* 1990; 211: 673-674)

When you are operating on a bleeding patient, it all comes down to a simple question: can you stop the bleeding before the patient runs out of blood? The key to success is not how you handle a vascular clamp, but, rather, how you handle yourself and your team. Bleeding control is not about mastering some cool moves. It is the ability to rapidly select appropriate hemostatic options and deploy them one after the other in a disciplined, effective fashion. Here's how to do it.

Choosing a hemostatic option

Don't reflexively jump on a bleeding vessel with the first available clamp. Instead, train yourself to think of every bleeding situation as a problem that requires an effective solution. There is always more than one alternative. Your job is to come up with a solution that will work for the specific situation in front of you. Therefore, the first rule of bleeding control is always select the simplest, most expedient hemostatic option.

Begin with the simplest hemostatic option

What are your options? If you have some surgical experience, your list must begin with "do nothing." This is often an excellent choice because relying on intrinsic hemostasis works surprisingly well for certain types of minor hemorrhage, like superficial oozing from solid organs. Your list of options probably goes on to electrocautery and ligation and then gradually escalates through the use of hemostatic sutures, packing, balloon tamponade, and all the way up to a formal vascular repair. You will not insert a hemostatic suture unless simpler means have either failed or are inappropriate. Therefore, the second underlying principle is a graded response.

Bleeding control is a graded response

If the first solution you chose didn't work, gradually escalate your efforts. An experienced surgeon rapidly zooms in on the 2-3 best hemostatic options for a given situation. This principle of a graded response has an important corollary: while you deploy a hemostatic solution, think ahead and prepare an alternative in case your selected technique doesn't work. Why is this important?

The more complex your next hemostatic solution, the more time it takes to prepare. When faced with massive bleeding from an inaccessible site, preparing an alternative becomes crucial. If your chosen solution doesn't work and you are not ready with an immediate alternative, you are up the creek in search of a paddle. Having a hemostatic option ready is not an accident. It requires careful planning and intimate familiarity with the equipment or tools you will need and where they can be found.

> **Be ready with an alternative hemostatic option**

Temporary and definitive control

Temporary control is like plugging a hole in a leaky bucket with your finger. Definitive control is fixing the bucket. In massive bleeding, temporary control is always the first step because it allows you to assess the situation and deploy an appropriate definitive hemostatic measure.

Temporary solutions must be quick, effective, and atraumatic. In certain situations, especially when the bleeder is either inaccessible or difficult to control, your temporary control maneuver (such as packing or balloon tamponade) may turn out to be the definitive measure because there is no better option. If you temporarily packed a badly injured liver and it stopped bleeding, don't remove the packs. You have achieved effective hemostasis - good enough. Move on.

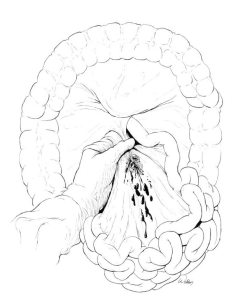

Obtaining temporary control

Manual or digital pressure is an excellent first choice. Control bleeding from a cardiac laceration with your finger. Pinch a mesenteric bleeder between thumb and forefinger. Compress a bleeding internal jugular vein with your finger. Insert a finger into a hosing groin wound.

Have your assistant compress an injured liver between the palms of both hands. Using your hands is quick, instinctive, completely atraumatic, and very effective.

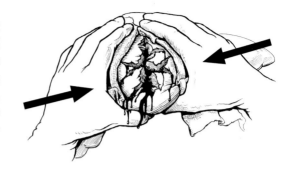

A classic error of the novice is to grab a clamp and try to blindly apply it in a pool of blood. This never works. Vascular clamps are effective when the target vessel has been dissected out and isolated, not when it has retracted into the tissue or is barely visible. Blind clamping is a sign of panic. You will not only fail to achieve control, but also will end up with an iatrogenic injury. Wild clamping of the descending thoracic aorta can easily result in an avulsed intercostal artery. A clamp applied hastily to the supraceliac aorta may perforate the esophagus. Blind clamping of a limb artery in a pool of blood will crush the adjacent nerve or injure the neighboring vein. Unless you are unusually talented, you cannot perforate the esophagus or crush the median nerve with your finger.

The finger is mightier than the clamp

Temporary packing is a good option for diffusely bleeding surfaces or cavities. It also frees your hands. However, packing will not control major arterial hemorrhage.

Pedicle control is another option. Does the injured organ have an immediately accessible vascular pedicle? The spleen, kidney and lung do, as does the bowel. One of the two vascular pedicles of the liver is easily accessible and can be rapidly pinched between thumb and forefinger or clamped with a non-crushing clamp, the famous Pringle maneuver. Similarly, if you mobilize the spleen or kidney you can rapidly control the pedicle with your fingers or a clamp. Twisting the lung upon itself is a simple and effective technique for hemorrhage control, as you will discover later (Chapter 11).

Temporary control buys you time. You can relax for just a moment, get the circulation back into your compressing hand, survey the situation and decide how to proceed.

Determine if the bleeding organ has a vascular pedicle

Small problem or BIG TROUBLE?

Now that you have gained temporary control and blood is no longer pouring all over your operative field, you have reached the key tactical decision in hemorrhage control: the distinction between a small problem and BIG TROUBLE.

A small problem is bleeding you can control using a direct hemostatic maneuver like clamping, suturing, or resecting the injured organ. Hemorrhage from an injured spleen is a small problem, as is a peripheral lung laceration or a low-grade liver injury. The great majority of bleeding situations you encounter during a trauma operation belong in this category.

BIG TROUBLE is an entirely different kettle of fish - a complex or inaccessible injury that poses a clear and immediate danger to your patient's life. A high-grade liver injury is the prototype of BIG TROUBLE. Bleeding from an iliac vein or a posterior intercostal artery deep in the lower chest are other examples.

The distinction between a small problem and BIG TROUBLE hinges on a combination of the bleeding rate and the accessibility of the bleeder. Several torn peripheral mesenteric vessels can bleed more than a contained hematoma in the base of the mesentery. Yet peripheral mesenteric bleeders are a small problem because they are accessible and easy to deal with. Bleeding from the root of the mesentery is BIG TROUBLE because it implies the need for vascular repair of an inaccessible superior mesenteric vessel.

The upper abdominal aorta is difficult to access and control; therefore, a midline supramesocolic hematoma is always BIG TROUBLE, regardless of how much it has bled. Free hemorrhage from the retrohepatic veins is BIG TROUBLE, not only because it is fast and furious, but also because you cannot get to it. Accessibility depends on the patient's position and on your incision. For example, an injury to the posterior thoracic wall may be inaccessible from an anterolateral thoracotomy incision, but easy to reach through a posterolateral thoracotomy.

Learn to distinguish between a small problem and BIG TROUBLE

Small problems and BIG TROUBLE require different mindsets and different operative approaches. You can tackle a small problem directly by immediately deploying appropriate hemostatic solutions until the bleeding stops. One of those solutions is likely to work, and the blood loss will be limited.

If you jump in and go head-to-head with BIG TROUBLE, you lose. The patient is profoundly hypotensive from massive blood loss. The OR team has no idea how bad the situation is or how you plan to deal with it. Exposure is bad. The 10-12 units of blood the patient will need are still in the blood bank. The vascular instruments you will need are stored outside the OR. In other words, the odds are overwhelmingly stacked against you and your patient even before you begin. A frontal attack (as you did for a small problem), will be like a bungee jump without a cord. Unless you do something to even the odds, you're finished before you start. So, what to do? The answer may surprise you.

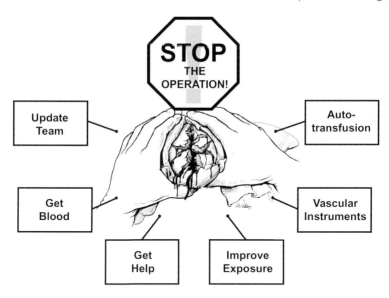

Once you have gained temporary control - STOP! Resist the temptation to immediately proceed to definitive control. Instead, organize and optimize your attack:

◆ Tell the anesthesiology team you are preparing for massive blood loss, urge them to catch up with volume replacement, and obtain at least 8-10 units of blood and a rapid infuser.
◆ Get an autotransfusion device primed and working.
◆ Have the OR team open and prepare vascular and thoracotomy instrument trays. Have the scrub nurse mount several polypropylene sutures (typically 3:0 - 5:0) on appropriate needle drivers.
◆ Determine your next 2-3 hemostatic options if you can. Will you need additional equipment like a Foley or Fogarty catheter? Will you need to improvise a balloon tamponade?
◆ Assess the capabilities of your OR team. Can they handle the roller-coaster ride ahead? Should you get additional help?
◆ Improve exposure by extending your incision, by inserting a self-retaining rotractor, or by rearranging your assistants.

While all these preparations are moving forward, don't fiddle with your temporary control. Leave the packs alone, maintain manual pressure, and don't move any clamps.

Don't fiddle - be a rock

Stand calmly and patiently with your hand on the bleeder and wait until the team is ready, the patient has been resuscitated, and the appropriate instruments and help are in the field. You have carefully set up your attack; now wage your battle under favorable circumstances.

When dealing with BIG TROUBLE, resist the temptation to keep on moving. The drama of exsanguinating hemorrhage is such that the team expects you to "do something." Stopping the operation in mid-air is the last thing they expect. Nevertheless, insist on completing all preparations even if it takes a considerable amount of time. We have occasionally stood with our hand on the bleeder for 15 minutes or more while the OR team completed preparations for battle and the patient was being resuscitated. Patience, preparation and planning give you a huge tactical advantage and dramatically improve your patient's chances.

We cannot overemphasize how critical it is to distinguish between a small problem and BIG TROUBLE. This may well be the most important decision of the entire operation. It is often a subjective decision that depends on your experience and confidence. A situation that a surgeon with limited trauma experience considers BIG TROUBLE may turn out to be a small problem for an experienced colleague. Nevertheless, if your impression is that the situation merits an organized attack, you will never go wrong by approaching it as BIG TROUBLE.

> **Always err on the side of caution**

Selected hemostatic techniques

Packing 101

Packing is one of the most underrated and badly taught techniques in trauma surgery. It is also one of your best weapons for dealing with BIG TROUBLE. Surgeons tend to think of packing as such an intuitive skill that they rarely bother to teach it properly. After all, you don't have to be a surgical genius to stuff some pieces of cloth around a bleeding liver - wrong!

The first rule of packing is to do it early. Since packing relies on clot formation, it can only be effective if done when the patient can still form good clots. Packing as a last resort, when the patient is coagulopathic and oozing from everywhere, is futile.

Pack early!

There are two main ways to pack. Packing *from without* is creating a sandwich. Packing *from within* is filling a cavity.

Pack from without by placing laparotomy pads outside the injured organ to reapproximate disrupted tissue planes. To achieve effective hemostasis you must create two opposing pressure vectors that compress the injured tissue between them; otherwise, your packing will not work. Effective packing is a sandwich, not a wrap.

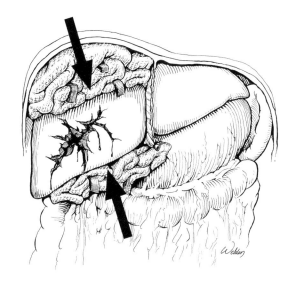

This technique is most often used in the injured liver. A good sandwich around the liver consists of two layers of laparotomy pads (above and below or anterior and posterior), approximating the disrupted tissue planes between them. These layers are supported, in turn, by the abdominal wall, the diaphragm, or by adjacent abdominal organs such as the stomach or large bowel. You cannot create a good sandwich by hanging two pieces of bread in mid-air. Your sandwich must make mechanical sense.

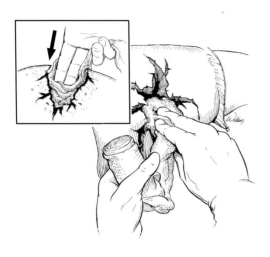

Packing from within is stuffing a crevice or an actively bleeding cavity with absorptive gauze. The filling, consisting of an unfolded gauze roll, is pushing outward against the walls of the injured parenchyma.

Your packing technique must be tailored to the shape of the injury. If dealing with a large bleeding surface or multiple injuries to a solid organ, pack from without. When packing a bleeding crevice, like the deep perineal wound of an open pelvic fracture, pack from within. In severe liver injuries, such as a stellate fracture of the dome of the right lobe, you will often find yourself using a combination of both techniques.

Packing from without or within works in opposite direction

The third rule of packing is to avoid overpacking. While constructing your sandwich around the injured liver, pay special attention to the patient's blood pressure. If it suddenly plummets and the anesthesiologist shows signs of distress, your packs may be compressing the inferior vena cava (IVC) and diminishing venous return to the heart. Carefully remove a few packs and reassess.

Too much packing is bad

The fourth (and last) rule of effective packing is to be paranoid. There is always the danger that your packs will not work, but it usually takes time to find out. Laparotomy pads have an amazing absorptive capacity, and the patient may well continue to bleed underneath them. If the patient's physiology allows, spend at least a few minutes doing something else, and then return to the packed area and re-examine it with very suspicious eyes. Is blood beginning to reaccumulate in the corners? Are the packs being slowly soaked? If you are not sure, peel off the most superficial layer of the sandwich and take a good look at the deeper layers. Are they turning pink and moist? If so, you have to take the sandwich apart because you do not have effective hemostasis. Never rely on the patient's clotting mechanism to compensate for ineffective packing. The best time to achieve hemostasis is before you leave the OR, not two hours (and 12 units of blood) later.

What if your packing doesn't work? First, remove the soaked packs one by one and inspect the injured area once more. Did you have a good sandwich solidly supported by surrounding structures, or did you build a "floating sandwich" in mid-air with no support? Do you need to add more packs? Should you add packing from within or from without? Is there an arterial bleeder in the injured area? If there is, you must deal with it directly using another hemostatic technique. Can you do something else to help stop the bleeding? Add a topical hemostatic agent? A blind hemostatic suture? Repack and wait again until you are sure that you have effective bleeding control.

Be paranoid about your packs

Inserting a blind hemostatic (figure of 8) suture

Use a blind hemostatic suture to control a bleeder that is either invisible or has retracted into the tissue. You cannot see the bleeder nor can you clamp and ligate it, but you can imagine where it is. After using blind hemostatic sutures so many times in elective and emergency surgery, you may feel confident that you know how to do it well. Chances are, you don't; here are some useful pointers:

◆ Make sure the anatomical situation is appropriate for a blind hemostatic suture. If the bleeding is close to an unexposed major vessel, always assume that the major vessel is the bleeder and expose it.

◆ Use a monofilament suture that will slide through the tissue rather than saw through it. Strange as it may seem, the key to success is not the suture, but the *size of the needle*. Choose the biggest needle that is appropriate for the situation.

◆ Place your first bite as close as possible to the site of bleeding. The purpose of this bite is not to achieve hemostasis, but to gain a good purchase on the tissue so you can lift it up by gently pulling on the suture with your non-dominant hand. Now you can see on which side of your first bite the bleeder is spurting. Your next bite will be for hemostasis, and since it is well-targeted, it will do useful work.

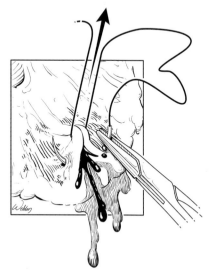

◆ If anyone ever bothered to teach you about blind hemostatic sutures, you probably know that your aim is to end up with a figure of 8 configuration that runs under the vessel proximally and distally to the bleeding site. This is nice in theory, but in practice you can never be sure in which direction the bleeding vessels lies. That's why they call it a blind stitch. Don't be disappointed if you end up needing more bites. It is okay to insert 3-4 bites instead of two, as long as the bites are close together and they work. We call this 4-bite suture a "figure of 16."

◆ Often, pulling on your blind suture will stop the bleeding. You must then decide if you wish to use it merely as a temporary hemostatic maneuver or tie it as a permanent solution. If you decide to tie it, remember to leave the ends long because you may wish to remove it later.

While inserting a blind stitch, plan your next hemostatic alternative. Experience has taught us that if you have not obtained hemostasis with four bites, you are not likely to achieve it with this stitch. Don't flail. Try something else.

The first bite of a hemostatic stitch gains purchase on the tissue

---

Aortic clamping

Aortic clamping is one of the traditional heroic maneuvers in trauma surgery. Use it either as an adjunct to resuscitation in a crashing patient or for global proximal control in major abdominal vascular trauma. You are unlikely to learn how to properly control the supraceliac abdominal aorta if you attempt it for the first time in a belly full of blood. Learn and practice the technique under elective circumstances.

Use aortic clamping judiciously, not reflexively. When used as a resuscitative adjunct, it temporarily corrects the numbers on the blood pressure monitor, but at the price of global visceral ischemia.

As with any major bleeding, the best immediately available tool is your hand. Pull the stomach downward and bluntly enter the lesser omentum in its avascular portion. Feel the aorta pulsating immediately below and to the right of the esophagus, and compress it against the spine. If you are occluding the aorta as a resuscitative maneuver, manual compression is often good enough. If you need formal aortic control, proceed with transabdominal supraceliac aortic clamping.

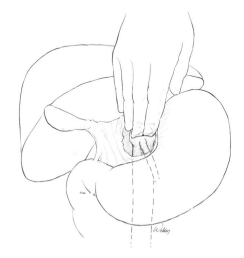

The key anatomical consideration in supraceliac clamping is that you are clamping the lowermost *thoracic* aorta, but doing it through the abdomen. As it emerges between the diaphragmatic crura, the aorta is enfolded by dense neural and fibrous tissue. In this particular aortic segment, it is difficult to obtain a good purchase with a clamp without dissecting around the aorta. Your best bet, therefore, is to go higher up, into the lower chest.

Clamp the lower thoracic aorta through the abdomen

If you have time, mobilize the left lateral lobe of the liver by incising the left triangular ligament. This improves your work space but is not essential to get to the aorta. Bluntly open the lesser omentum immediately to the right of the lesser curve of the stomach, and insert a Deaver retractor into the hole. Retraction of the stomach and duodenum to the left exposes the posterior peritoneum of the lesser sac and, underneath it, the right crus of the diaphragm.

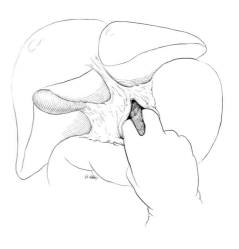

Palpate the pulsating aorta above the superior border of the pancreas to orient yourself. Bluntly make a hole in the posterior peritoneum; then, using either your finger or blunt-tipped Mayo scissors, separate the two limbs of the right crus of the diaphragm to expose the anterior wall of the lowermost thoracic aorta.

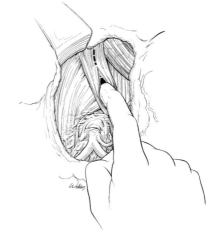

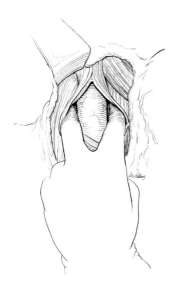

Using the fingers of your left hand, create just enough space on both sides of the aorta to accommodate a clamp. That is all the dissection you need. Take an aortic clamp and guide it to the correct position using the fingers of your left hand as a guide. Clamp, and check the distal aorta for pulsation.

The aortic clamp tends to fall forward into the wound. Encircle it with an umbilical tape and secure the tape to the drape over the patient's lower chest to immobilize the clamp. You are done.

THE KEY POINTS

▶   Begin with the simplest hemostatic option.

▶   Bleeding control is a graded response.

▶   Be ready with an alternative hemostatic option.

▶   The finger is mightier than the clamp.

▶   Determine if the bleeding organ has a vascular pedicle.

▶   Learn to distinguish between a small problem and BIG TROUBLE.

▶   Don't fiddle - be a rock.

▶   Always err on the side of caution.

▶   Pack early!

▶   Packing from without or within works in opposite direction.

▶   Too much packing is bad.

▶   Be paranoid about your packs.

▶   The first bite of a hemostatic stitch gains purchase on the tissue.

▶   Clamp the lower thoracic aorta through the abdomen.

Chapter 3
Your Vascular Toolkit

*Human beings, who are almost unique in having the
ability to learn from the experience of others, are also
remarkable for their apparent disinclination to do so*

~ Douglas Adams

Imagine yourself preparing to repair a gunshot injury to the femoral artery. The 29-year-old patient has an arteriovenous fistula just below the right groin. You feel a strong thrill and hear a bruit, definitely what our residents call "a great case."

You have a small problem: no angiogram of the injured area. Come to think of it, you have neither heparin nor monofilament suture. You don't even have a proper vascular clamp. Your great case is rapidly becoming a nightmare. How would you feel if the only vascular tools you had were some fine cotton sutures on straight needles and a pair of crude non-crushing clamps? Can you imagine grabbing a scalpel and just going for the injured vessel? This is exactly what J.B. Murphy, an amazing Chicago surgeon, did in 1897. He fixed a femoral arteriovenous fistula armed only with a detailed knowledge of the anatomy, years of practicing vascular repairs in the laboratory, and sheer guts. The operation took 2.5 hours and went smoothly with no complications.

More than a hundred years later, you have a dazzling array of vascular instruments at your disposal when facing major vascular trauma. But you cannot zoom in on a lacerated popliteal artery and forget that it belongs to a critically injured patient who also has a fractured pelvis, a contused lung, and possibly an intracranial hemorrhage.

This chapter will first acquaint you with useful general principles to guide you when coming face-to-face with a vascular injury. We assume you are familiar with basic vascular techniques and will show you how to adapt them to the trauma situation. Second, we will present a useful toolkit of technical options for damage control and definitive repair of vascular injuries. Remember, a good outcome in vascular trauma depends more on clear thinking and keeping priorities straight than on cool gadgets and elegant moves. Keep your vascular toolkit in mind as you learn to deal with specific vascular injuries in subsequent chapters.

Sequence and priorities

Much like any other trauma operation, avoid making "exciting discoveries" when dealing with major vascular injuries by following a well-defined sequence of steps.

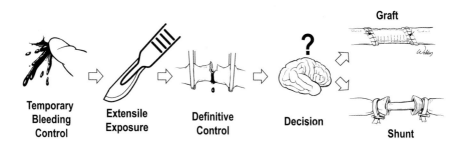

Temporary Bleeding Control ⇨ **Extensile Exposure** ⇨ **Definitive Control** ⇨ **Decision** ⇨ **Graft** / **Shunt**

Bleeding and ischemia, the two manifestations of vascular trauma, represent different priorities. A bleeding carotid artery is an immediate threat to the patient's life, and you must control it NOW! Not so with an ischemic leg from a superficial femoral artery injury, where you have a window of several hours to save the leg. This is why bleeding is part of the ABC of the primary survey of the injured patient, while ischemia isn't.

Bleeding and ischemia are different priorities

Control external bleeding

Obtain initial control of external hemorrhage by simple digital or manual pressure. If possible, rapidly transfer responsibility for compressing the bleeding vessel to an assistant, and prep the hand as part of the operative field. Your assistant can then continue to apply pressure while you make an incision proximal to (or around) the compressing hand to expose the injured vessel.

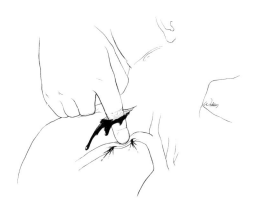

Use a balloon catheter when the bleeding source is deep and the wound is narrow (e.g. bullet wound), especially in transition zones between the trunk and the limbs, such as the groin, supraclavicular fossa, axilla, or neck. In these locations, manual compression is less effective. Insert a Foley catheter into the bleeding tract, inflate the balloon until bleeding stops, and then clamp the main port of the Foley. If the wound is wide and the balloon pops out, approximate the wound edges around it with a stitch to help hold it in place.

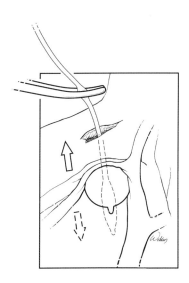

Balloon tamponade controls external bleeding in transition zones

Before you begin

Do not begin a vascular exploration without complete knowledge of the patient's trauma burden. How much time has passed since the injury? How much has the patient bled? How urgent is the brain contusion? What is the plan for the fracture in the extremity you are operating on? You must incorporate all this information into your decision-making or you will end up with an awesome vascular reconstruction - in a dead patient.

Know the patient's total trauma burden and physiology

Proper sequencing is a huge factor in peripheral vascular trauma because injuries to limbs typically also involve bones, nerves and soft tissue. As a general rule, bone alignment comes before vascular repair. Fixing fractures involves such fun activities as hammering, rimming and chiseling, moving bones, and other tricks that a 5:0 suture line does not tolerate very well. So, if the limb is not grossly ischemic and the planned orthopedic procedure is short (e.g. external fixation), let the orthopedic surgeon do it before the vascular exploration. If the limb is grossly ischemic or if the injury is actively bleeding, you have to go first. Control the injured artery, insert a temporary shunt, and do a fasciotomy to increase the tolerance of the limb to ischemia. Let the orthopedic surgeon achieve bone alignment, and only then do the definitive vascular repair on a stable extremity.

Align bone before arterial reconstruction

Angiography

Preoperative angiography is not an option for a hemodynamically unstable or actively bleeding patient. In a stable patient, get an angiogram if you can, especially if you aren't sure where the injury is. Consider a patient with multiple gunshot wounds or several fractures in the same extremity. How will you know where the injury is without a road map? With a single penetrating injury, things are simpler because you can find the injury with a limited exploration, so you can skip the angiogram.

Depending on your experience and the local circumstances, you have three options for obtaining an angiogram:

1. A single-shot angiogram performed in the ER - rapidly becoming a lost art.
2. A formal study performed in the angiography suite or OR - endovascular intervention could preclude the need for open repair.
3. Intraoperative angiography by cannulation of the exposed artery - best results are obtained by clamping the inflow before injecting the dye.

Get an angiogram if the patient is stable

Pre-emptive fasciotomy

Consider doing a fasciotomy *before* beginning the vascular repair, not when compartment syndrome is clinically obvious. When operating on an ischemic extremity, you often know that the formal repair is going to take time. Your safest course of action is to do a pre-emptive fasciotomy.

A popliteal artery repair is a good example. Regardless of your experience, popliteal reconstructions always end up taking longer than you expected. The unforgiving nature of these injuries and the paucity of collaterals around the knee virtually guarantee you will not finish this operation without a fasciotomy. Be smart. Do it before the vascular reconstruction.

We do a four-compartment fasciotomy using a double incision technique. Place your lateral incision approximately two fingerbreadths lateral to the edge of the tibia. Open the fascia all the way down to the ankle; then, identify and incise the intermuscular septum separating the anterior and lateral compartments. Avoid damage to the lateral peroneal nerve that lies in close proximity to the head of the fibula. Then, make a medial incision approximately a fingerbreadth behind the medial edge of the tibial shaft. Injury to the greater saphenous vein is not part of this incision, so be careful. Using the cautery, detach the soleus muscle from the medial aspect of the tibia to decompress the deep posterior compartment.

> **Do pre-emptive fasciotomy before popliteal artery repair**

Extensile exposure and key landmarks

The fundamental principle of vascular exploration is extensile exposure, which means that you must be able to extend your incision proximally or distally along the same axis as the original incision. The obvious examples are lower extremity incisions along the medial aspect of the leg. Using these incisions, exposure of the superficial femoral, popliteal, and tibial vessels can easily be extended into each other.

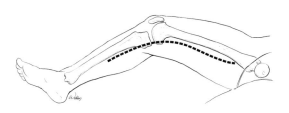

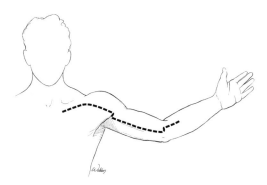

In the upper extremity, subclavian, axillary and brachial exposures are similarly extensile. Avoid non-extensile exposures, such as the posterior approach to the popliteal vessels or the transaxillary approach to the axillary artery, because they limit your access and restrict your options.

When dissecting an injured vessel, it is easy to get lost. The broken bones, bleeding muscle, and torn vessels are a minefield, even for an experienced vascular surgeon. Safe dissection in hostile territory hinges on the use of key anatomical landmarks to help you orient yourself and identify your target. In the lower extremity, key landmarks are the bones (femur and tibia), because the neurovascular bundle is located immediately behind it. Find the posterior aspect of the femur or tibia, and you have found the femoral or posterior tibial artery, respectively. The pectoralis minor is your key landmark when looking for the axillary vessels, as is the median nerve when exposing the brachial artery. You will find many examples of the use of key anatomical landmarks throughout this book because it is an extremely useful concept when you're in trouble in unfamiliar territory.

Know the key anatomical landmarks

Proximal control and anatomical barriers

What is definitive vascular control? It is the accurate placement of vascular clamps (or other atraumatic means of occlusion) across the inflow and outflow tracts of an injured vessel. Proximal control is key. Entering a hematoma without first obtaining proximal control away from the site of injury is a stupid mistake that often leads to excessive blood loss, disorganized fumbling, panic, iatrogenic injury, and sometimes exsanguination.

Prevent your dissection from becoming a "search and destroy mission," by obtaining proximal control outside the hematoma that surrounds the injury. Begin in virgin territory where tissue planes are normal, and gradually advance toward the injured segment

Experienced surgeons go beyond *anatomical barriers* to get proximal control. Yes, you guessed it - another key concept. Many anatomical structures serve as barriers to the expansion of hematoma. Consider the inguinal ligament in penetrating injuries to the groin. Below the ligament you will find only blood, sweat, and tears. Above it, you are in virgin territory where you can easily isolate and control the external iliac artery. The pericardium is, similarly, a barrier to the expansion of a mediastinal hematoma, and the diaphragm blocks the extension of a midline retroperitoneal hematoma. Go to the other side of anatomical barriers to find easy proximal control.

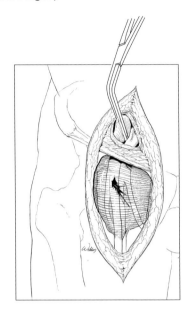

A useful option for proximal control in the limbs, often forgotten in the heat of battle, is a pneumatic tourniquet on the upper arm or proximal thigh. Using it saves blood and simplifies the dissection. Once you have isolated and clamped the injured vessels, deflate the tourniquet.

Get proximal control outside the hematoma

Distal control

How important is distal control? It depends. Usually proximal control alone does not dry up the operative field because back bleeding from the distal vessel continues to give you grief. The patient will not exsanguinate, but you will not be able to do a vascular reconstruction in peace.

For the aorta and its proximal branches (e.g. subclavian and common iliac arteries), proximal clamping serves only to convert fierce audible bleeding into weaker bleeding, but you still cannot see the injury well, and the patient is losing blood at an alarming rate. You must obtain distal control. Do this outside the hematoma if you can. If not, expose the injury under proximal control, and gain distal control from within the hematoma. Typical locations where distal control is difficult are the distal internal carotid artery, subclavian artery and the large veins of the pelvis.

For distal control from within the hematoma, choose the technique that makes the most tactical sense. Can you rapidly dissect the distal vessel and clamp it? Apply a side-biting clamp? Insert an intraluminal balloon catheter (typically a Fogarty catheter connected to a 3-way stopcock) into the outflow tract? This last technique, frequently used in elective vascular surgery, allows you to gain distal control without having to dissect out the distal vessel.

> **Use an intraluminal balloon for problematic distal control**

Exploring the injured vessel

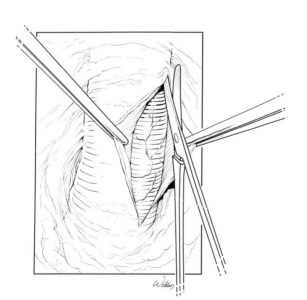

Your safe dissection plane along an artery is the periadventitial plane directly on the arterial wall. It will carry you safely from uninjured territory to the injured segment without lacerating the vessel or ripping off branches. You know you are in this safe plane when you see the pearly-white arterial wall with the vasa-vasorum on it.

As you enter the hematoma, define the injury by rapidly answering three questions:

- Which vessels are involved? Artery, vein, or both?
- How bad is it? Laceration or complete transection?
- Where are you? Are there major branches, joints, or other structures nearby?

You cannot assess an arterial injury by external inspection. This is especially true in blunt trauma, where the artery may appear intact on the outside yet hide a disrupted intima on the inside. You must open the artery and define the extent of intimal damage. With few exceptions, your arteriotomy will be longitudinal. Make sure you see the full length of the intimal damage.

Once you have defined the injury, carefully debride the injured wall back to healthy tissue. Don't compromise on intima that looks "almost normal" or is "slightly bruised," because you are buying yourself and your patient early postoperative thrombosis. There are no grey areas here - the intima is either healthy or it's not.

Define the full extent of the vascular injury

Developing a work space

Remember that you are not exploring the injured vessel just to have a look at it. You are going to work on it, and you need a work space. A laparotomy or thoracotomy automatically provides you with an open cavity that is your work space. In the extremities and the neck, there are no ready-made cavities, so you have to carve one out.

Develop your work space in stages. First, make the incision. Then, deepen it into the subcutaneous tissue and incise the deep fascia. Insert a self-retaining retractor and continue your dissection to isolate the neurovascular bundle using the key landmarks. As you make progress, continuously reassess your emerging work space. Is the incision long enough? Should you relocate the self-retaining retractor to a deeper plane? Should the corner of the wound be manually retracted? Do you have enough space on both sides of the artery to sew conveniently? Can you bring the vessel more toward you (make it more superficial) by mobilizing it? The more you invest in optimizing your work space, the more time you will save during the reconstruction. When called to assist in a vascular trauma case, our first move is to extend the incision and optimize the work space.

Gradually develop and optimize your work space

The key strategic decision

Now it's time for your strategic decision, the choice between vascular damage control and definitive repair - a simple enough concept, but often a tough decision.

First, consider the type of repair required. Formal vascular repairs come in two flavors: simple and complex. A simple repair is a single, short suture line that can be completed quickly, even under adverse circumstances. If such a lateral repair will work - just do it.

A *complex repair* is a vascular anastomosis (or more than one). An end-to-end anastomosis, a patch angioplasty and an interposition graft are complex repairs. They take time to set up and perform but do you have the time? First, consider the patient's physiology. There is no point in doing an interposition graft in a coagulopathic patient who will just bleed on and on from the suture lines. This patient needs to be in the intensive care unit, rewarmed and resuscitated, not on the operating table losing more blood and becoming progressively hypothermic. You must bail out.

Second, consider additional factors. Is the patient unstable or actively bleeding in another cavity? If the answer is yes, damage control is your only option. Do you have the experience required? Can you get adequate help? Are the necessary vascular instruments at hand? If the answer to any of these questions is no, again choose damage control.

Decide between complex vascular repair and damage control

Vascular damage control techniques

The two major damage control techniques for vascular trauma are ligation and shunt insertion.

Ligation

Ligation of an injured vessel is often a no brainer. The external carotid artery, celiac axis, and internal iliac artery are obvious examples of arteries that can be ligated with impunity. Other arteries, such as the subclavian or brachial, can be ligated with a low risk of limb-threatening ischemia. If you are forced to bail out but plan to repair the vessel later, don't ligate it - use a temporary shunt instead.

Most large veins can be ligated with impunity or with acceptable consequences (such as leg edema). In the past, repair of the popliteal vein was viewed as crucial for a good outcome with popliteal artery reconstruction, but this sacred cow was slaughtered long ago. There are even reports of successful ligation of the portal vein, although this is probably one of the very few visceral veins that you should repair if you can. Remember, ligating a vessel is not an admission of defeat; it can be a sign of good judgment.

Ligation is not an admission of defeat

Temporary shunts

If you have little vascular experience or are operating in austere circumstances, a temporary shunt may be your best option. Insert a shunt when the patient's physiology is prohibitive, when orthopedic alignment of the bones precedes the arterial repair, or when you lack the resources to do a complex reconstruction.

Shunt material is not an issue; use whatever is immediately available. We have successfully used pieces of nasogastric tubes, suction catheters, carotid shunts, and silastic T-tubes. We prefer to use an Argyle shunt (pediatric chest tube) because we use it regularly in carotid surgery, and it is easy to handle. However, in one of the most spectacular cases of successful shunting that we have seen, a military surgeon in the field used a segment of nasogastric tube to shunt a transected femoral artery in the groin.

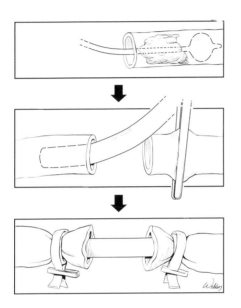

Insert the shunt using a well-defined sequence of steps. Begin by clearing the inflow and outflow tracts of the injured artery with a Fogarty catheter, if available. If not, gently squeeze the proximal and distal ends of the transected artery to express clot, and release the clamps momentarily to flush out both inflow and outflow. Choose a shunt of the largest diameter that will fit comfortably in the vessel, trimming it to the desired length. Gently insert it into the distal, then proximal artery (since backflow is easier to control than foreflow). Now, fix the shunt in place. The simplest technique is to secure the shunt to the artery proximally and distally with heavy silk ties. However, this is traumatic to the arterial wall and will later require additional debridement of the artery beyond the ligature line when you remove the shunt. Our preference is to pass a vessel loop twice around the shunted artery and gently cinch it with a large metal clip or a Rummel tourniquet. Now, assess the distal perfusion by listening for a Doppler signal over the outflow artery. You're done.

Shunt failure shortly after insertion is due to one of the following:

◆   Inadequate inflow (proximal injury or residual thrombus).
◆   Compromised outflow (residual clot or migration of the shunt into a distal arterial branch).

◆ Obstructed shunt (angulation due to excessive length or ligatures that are too tight).

◆ Shunt dislodgement (presents as a rapidly expanding hematoma).

Clear the inflow and outflow tracts before shunt insertion

Definitive repair techniques

You have three options for definitive repair: end-to-end anastomosis, patch angioplasty, or interposition graft. An end-to-end anastomosis sounds like an excellent choice because it involves only a single straightforward suture line. Unfortunately, with experience you will find yourself using this solution less frequently than you think. In young patients, the ends of transected arteries retract a surprising distance, creating a large gap. The inexperienced surgeon will spend time mobilizing both ends of the transected artery in a heroic effort to bring them together. This entails additional dissection and sacrificing branches along the way. Despite these efforts, the resulting end-to-end anastomosis will often be under considerable tension and will have to be redone, this time using an interposition graft. Therefore, in vascular trauma, the best option for complete transection of an artery is often an interposition graft.

Transected artery = interposition graft

Patch angioplasty is an option to keep in mind, especially if at least half the circumference of the artery is still intact or if the vessel is small. We rarely repair a laceration in a brachial or popliteal artery without a small vein patch, because even a transversely oriented lateral repair will narrow the lumen of these small vessels.

Before you begin the repair, pass a Fogarty catheter proximally and distally, and then flush the vessel with heparinized saline. The Fogarty catheter will not only evacuate clot, but also will dilate a spastic vessel, facilitating your repair.

Systemic heparin has a bad reputation in vascular trauma, raising fears of causing bleeding in the adjacent traumatized soft tissue or in remote injuries. However, when dealing with an isolated arterial injury, especially if your repair is going to take time, give systemic heparin to protect the distal microcirculation. Popliteal artery repairs are a good example where systemic heparin makes a difference.

Do you have to repair injured veins? It is a luxury, not a must. If a vein injury requires a complex repair, it may not be worth the trouble. These repairs are technically more demanding than arterial reconstructions, often with inferior long-term patency, and may be unnecessary. If the patient has other injuries that require attention, sustained a significant physiological insult, or has been in the OR for many hours, ligate the injured vein without hesitation.

If you decide to indulge in a combined arterial and venous repair, the venous reconstruction should come first because a thrombosed vein cannot be effectively cleared. Remember to interpose viable soft tissue between the venous and arterial repairs to prevent a fistula.

Vein repair is a luxury - not a must

Working with grafts

Choice of graft material is a major controversy in vascular trauma. No one would consider a synthetic graft below the knee or distal to the shoulder because the vessels are too small; 4mm synthetic grafts simply don't work. This focuses the controversy on the femoral artery. The proponents of vein grafts emphasize how well they work, although there is no good evidence that they do better than synthetic grafts in young patients with intact outflow tracts. The proponents of synthetic grafts emphasize how well they *fail*, since, in the presence of infection and exposure, a vein graft dessicates and dissolves, resulting in sudden hemorrhage. A synthetic graft fails gradually by forming a pseudoaneurysm. Another advantage of the synthetic graft is expediency. Our personal preference is synthetic graft for femoral artery reconstruction. The truth is that it does not matter which material you use, as long as you do it well.

Graft protection is a cardinal principle in vascular trauma. When planning your reconstruction, remember that an interposition graft in a traumatized and contaminated field invites disaster. You have to route the graft through a clean field or cover it with well-vascularized soft tissue. Graft protection considerations may dictate the operative sequence: bowel repair and peritoneal toilet before an abdominal vascular reconstruction; soft tissue debridement before an interposition graft in an injured extremity. Occasionally, you may have to improvise an unconventional extra-anatomic route for the graft to avoid either a heavily contaminated environment or a large soft tissue defect.

Vascular trauma is essentially the art of dealing with young arteries that are soft, pliable, and easily undergo vasoconstriction. Remember these inherent qualities when sewing in a graft. The technical principle of driving the needle always from inside the artery out, so religiously taught in elective vascular surgery, is irrelevant in vascular trauma. You won't raise an intimal flap in a healthy artery, even if you go from outside in. So, work in whatever direction is most convenient, but always have tremendous respect for the arterial wall, because it will not forgive bad passage of the needle or jerking the suture sideways. The trajectory of the needle must always be perpendicular to the arterial wall.

Do not injure the artery with your vascular instruments. Pass a Fogarty catheter only a few centimeters above and below the injury, and do not over-inflate, or you will denude the healthy intima. Close the jaws of a vascular clamp gently ("only two clicks") so as not to crush the artery.

A major pitfall with young arteries is size mismatch. It is easy to insert too small a graft into a vasoconstricted artery, only to later realize you have created a bottleneck that invites early failure. This is particularly common in the aorta and iliac arteries of young adults. Because the vasoconstricted aorta will dilate later, make a conscious decision to select a slightly larger graft than what you deem necessary at the moment.

> **Vascular trauma is the art of dealing with healthy arteries**

THE KEY POINTS

▶ Bleeding and ischemia are different priorities.

▶ Balloon tamponade controls external bleeding in transition zones.

▶ Know the patient's total trauma burden and physiology,

▶ Align bone before arterial reconstruction.

▶ Get an angiogram if the patient is stable.

▶ Do pre-emptive fasciotomy before popliteal artery repair.

▶ Know the key anatomical landmarks.

▶ Get proximal control outside the hematoma.

▶ Use an intraluminal balloon for problematic distal control.

▶ Define the full extent of the vascular injury.

▶ Gradually develop and optimize your work space.

▶ Decide between complex vascular repair and damage control.

▶ Ligation is not an admission of defeat.

▶ Clear the inflow and outflow tracts before shunt insertion.

▶ Transected artery = interposition graft.

▶ Vein repair is a luxury - not a must.

▶ Vascular trauma is the art of dealing with healthy arteries.

Chapter 4
The Crash Laparotomy

Damn the torpedoes, full speed ahead!

~ Admiral David J. Farragut

In most surgical training programs, you spend much time in the OR with the cautery in hand, merrily blasting away at stray erythrocytes while your teacher unobtrusively opens the correct tissue planes with a right-angled clamp, an ever-present sucker tip or an educated finger, pretending you are doing the case. The way you cut tissue, tie knots, arrange retraction, and suture bowel are all part of the technical language of general surgery.

A trauma operation is not an accelerated version of the elective procedure. It requires a different technical language and, most importantly, a different mindset. In this chapter, we demonstrate these differences by taking a familiar operation, exploratory laparotomy, and translating it into the technical language of trauma surgery. Rapid alternations between swift, crude exposure maneuvers and meticulous dissection are the hallmarks of a trauma laparotomy. It's like dancing through a real minefield while playing DOOM™ on your laptop. Get the picture?

The operative sequence

Every trauma laparotomy follows the same methodical, practiced operative sequence.

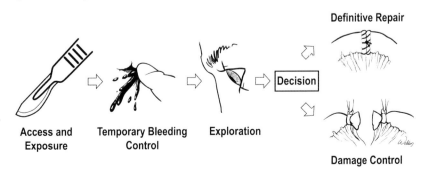

Access and Exposure   Temporary Bleeding Control   Exploration   Decision   Definitive Repair   Damage Control

The key decision in this algorithm is the choice between definitive repair and damage control. The earlier you make this decision, the better for the patient.

Gaining access

Enter the peritoneal cavity through a long midline incision, the Texas name for which is "Hey diddle diddle, right down the middle." The less stable the patient, the faster you should dive in. Take the scalpel and make a bold cut through the skin and subcutaneous tissue. If you grab the diathermy to systematically barbeque subcutaneous bleeders in a patient with a systolic pressure of 60, you are probably in the wrong specialty and should consider a career change. The hypotensive trauma patient is peripherally vasoconstricted, and you are wasting time on nonsense oozing while rapid intra-abdominal bleeding continues unabated 2cm below the tip of your diathermy. Sounds pretty stupid because it is.

The incision begins below the xiphoid, skirts around the umbilicus, and ends above the pubis. An experienced surgeon uses three long and precise passes of the knife to enter the peritoneal cavity. The first sweep gets you past the skin and into the subcutaneous tissue. The second pass lands you on the linea alba. Develop the ability to gauge the depth of the subcutaneous fat and the "feel" of landing on the fascia without cutting it. The third and last pass of the knife divides the linea alba to visualize the preperitoneal fat.

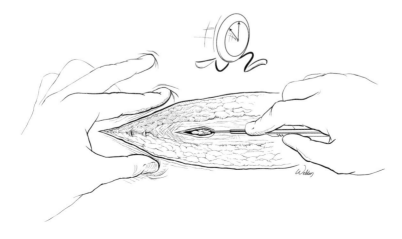

Train yourself to make the incision like a pro. If it takes you five or six sweeps, you are okay but not yet ready for prime time.

The key maneuver is to cut in the midline where the abdominal wall is thinnest and entry into the abdomen is quickest. This is called "gaining the midline." A good marker of the midline is the decussation of the fibers of the anterior rectus sheath. If you see muscle underneath your fascial incision, steer medially.

Now, take advantage of a little-known anatomical fact. In most patients, the peritoneum just cranial to the umbilicus is either very thin or has a defect. There is only very thin preperitoneal fat in this area, making it the ideal spot for entering the peritoneal cavity. Forget the elaborate dance (often taught in elective surgery) of picking up 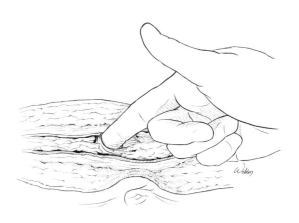 the peritoneum between two pairs of pickups and making a small nick to let air in. Simply poke a finger into this peritoneal defect immediately above the umbilicus, and you find yourself in the peritoneal cavity.

Using a pair of heavy scissors, cut the peritoneum, together with the overlying preperitoneal fat, to the full extent of the incision. Use your non-dominant hand to push the intestines down to protect them from your advancing scissors. Identify the falciform ligament and divide it between clamps to gain access to the right upper quadrant. You're in the belly, ready to Rock n' Roll.

Enter the belly with three sweeps of the knife and one educated finger

A word of caution

The major pitfall during a crash laparotomy is iatrogenic injury. The left lateral lobe of the liver, the small bowel, and the bladder are in jeopardy in the upper, middle, and lower parts of the incision, respectively. On a particularly bad day or if you are especially gifted, you can injure all three organs in one bold sweep.

If the patient has a pelvic fracture, entering a pelvic hematoma is generally considered a bad move. Make an upper midline incision, carefully peek into the abdomen, and extend your incision downward below the umbilicus under direct vision.

Entering the abdomen through a previous laparotomy scar can be time-consuming and exasperating in a hypotensive patient. The safe technique is to extend the incision beyond the old scar into virgin territory and enter the peritoneal cavity where adhesions are less likely. Then, open the old scar piecemeal, after making sure that the undersurface is clear and pushing adherent loops of bowel out of the way. Even if you have completed your incision without mishap, you may still face adhesions of bowel loops to the anterior abdominal wall. When these adhesions are dense or multiple, you will feel a little stupid engaging in careful adhesiolysis while the anesthesiologist is pumping unit after unit of blood into your hypotensive patient. Is there a quicker way in? Yes, there is.

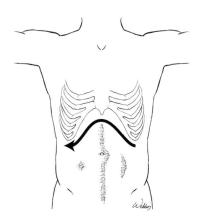

A creative solution in an abdomen with multiple old scars would be not to enter in the midline, but make a bilateral subcostal incision (also known as a Double Kocher or a rooftop incision). The incision itself takes longer to make and close, but you will more than make up for it by skirting around the troublesome midline adhesions.

Stay away from old scars

Once inside the abdomen

When you first peek into the open abdomen, all you can see is a spaghetti of bowel loops swimming in a pool of blood and clots. Your first priorities are to achieve temporary hemostasis and evacuate the blood so you can see what is going on.

The key maneuver now is *evisceration*. Rapidly gather the small bowel loops outside the abdomen toward you (to the right and up). Don't just shove laparotomy pads into the open abdomen without eviscerating the bowel, an act akin to throwing paper napkins into a bowel of soup - and a total waste of time.

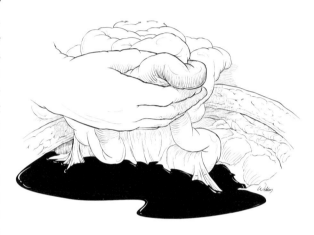

Evisceration converts the bloody mess into a manageable work space, allowing you to see what you are doing. Rapidly evacuate the blood and achieve temporary hemostasis.

Eviscerate the bowel early

Choose a temporary hemostatic technique based on the mechanism of injury. In blunt trauma, begin with empirical packing. Hand your assistant a large retractor to elevate the abdominal wall of each quadrant in turn, and pack the abdomen rapidly. Begin with the right upper quadrant by placing your left hand over the dome of the liver, pulling it gently toward you, and placing packs over your hand above and then below the liver. Pack the right paracolic gutter. Move to the left and put your non-dominant hand above the spleen, pulling it gently toward you, then pack over your retracting hand above the spleen and left lobe of the liver. Create a sandwich by packing medial to the spleen. Move to the left paracolic gutter and then to the pelvis, and pack them. All this time, the eviscerated bowel remains out of the way. If blood is accumulating on the eviscerated bowel, the source is a mesenteric bleeder. Deal with it directly. During packing and while your non-

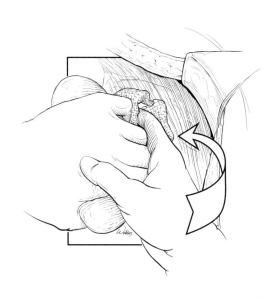

dominant hand is retracting and protecting the liver and spleen, feel for any obvious injury, and begin planning your approach based on this tactile assessment.

Empirical abdominal packing does not arrest major arterial hemorrhage. It gives you time to organize your effort and divides the peritoneal cavity into several distinct areas you can explore systematically. Packing works well in blunt trauma because the most likely sources of hemorrhage are the liver, spleen and mesentery. Bleeding from most solid organ injuries can be temporarily controlled with local pressure, while mesenteric injuries are immediately apparent in the eviscerated bowel loops.

In blunt trauma, begin with empirical packing

In penetrating trauma, your best bet is to go straight at the bleeder. Glance into the eviscerated peritoneal cavity to determine where the bleeding is coming from. You will then be able to achieve targeted rather than blind temporary hemostasis. Pack a bleeding solid organ or a contained retroperitoneal hematoma. Manually compress a freely bleeding vessel. Clamp a mesenteric bleeder. Some surgeons pack empirically in penetrating trauma cases, just as they do in blunt trauma. We prefer to see exactly what is bleeding and address it directly.

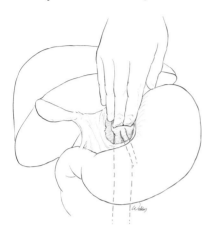

In an exsanguinating patient, consider compressing the aorta. Manual compression of the supraceliac aorta through a hole in the lesser omentum is much safer and as effective as formal clamping. Transfer responsibility for aortic compression to the right hand of your assistant.

> **In penetrating trauma, eviscerate and go for the bleeder**

Surveying the battlefield

Once major bleeding is temporarily controlled, rapidly explore the abdomen. The transverse colon extends across the middle of your incision, and its mesentery divides the peritoneal cavity into two visceral compartments. The supramesocolic compartment contains the liver, stomach, and spleen. The inframesocolic compartment contains the small bowel, colon, bladder, and female reproductive organs.

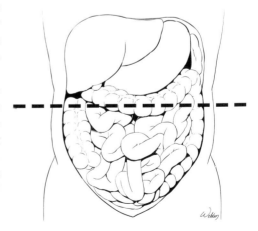

Systematically explore the peritoneal cavity. It doesn't matter where you begin as long as you maintain a linear sequence that covers the entire content of both compartments. This sequence should be routine and reproducible. You learn it in residency and methodically repeat it in subsequent operations, in your sleep (and in court).

Begin your exploration of the inframesocolic compartment by lifting the transverse colon cranially and running the gut from the ligament of Treitz down to the rectum (or from the rectum backwards to the ligament of Treitz).

Two pairs of hands - yours and your assistant's - flip each loop of bowel in a coordinated fashion to inspect both sides, paying special attention to the mesentery. The posterior aspect of the transverse colon and the hepatic and splenic flexures are notorious for missed injuries. If you identify a bowel perforation, control the spillage with a soft bowel clamp. You typically smell a colonic perforation before you see it. Remember to look at the bladder and female reproductive organs in the pelvis.

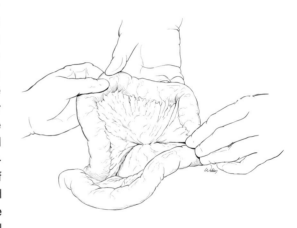

Pull the transverse colon caudad to explore the supramesocolic compartment. Inspect and palpate the liver and gallbladder, and palpate the right kidney. Then, inspect the stomach all the way up to the esophagogastric (EG) junction and the duodenum (including what you can see of the duodenal loop). To fully visualize the duodenum, you must do a Kocher maneuver and take down the ligament of Treitz. Palpate the convexity of the spleen and the left kidney. Don't forget to inspect both hemidiaphragms and note any injury, as well as whether the diaphragm is flat or bulging into the abdomen.

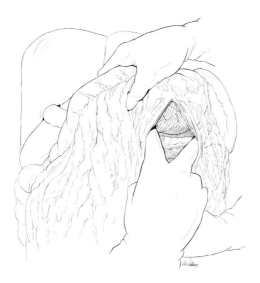

Next, explore the lesser sac. As your assistant holds up the stomach and transverse colon, pulling them apart to stretch the greater omentum, go to the left side of the omentum (it is typically less vascular), and bluntly poke a hole in it. This allows a good look at the posterior wall of the stomach and the body and tail of the pancreas.

Explore the supramesocolic and inframesocolic compartments

So far, you have explored the peritoneal cavity. Underneath, the retroperitoneum, a separate visceral compartment, is still lurking in the dark.

Exploring the retroperitoneum

To get to the retroperitoneal structures, you must go *behind* the intraperitoneal organs. Global exposure of the entire retroperitoneum is impossible, so the key principle is limited exposure of the relevant retroperitoneal structures by rotating the overlying intraperitoneal organs medially.

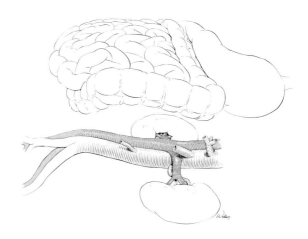

Decide which retroperitoneal structure you wish to explore, guided by clinical suspicion that it may be injured. Your clinical suspicion is based on the trajectory of the wounding missile or on the presence of a retroperitoneal hematoma. For example, any hematoma or blood staining around the duodenal loop mandates mobilization of the second part of the duodenum and the head of the pancreas. Penetrating injury to the ascending or descending colon requires mobilization of the entire injured side of the colon to examine not only its posterior wall, but also the adjacent ureter. How can you get the intraperitoneal organs off the underlying retroperitoneum? By doing a medial visceral rotation.

Keep retroperitoneal exploration targeted and limited

Left-sided medial visceral rotation (Mattox maneuver)

The least accessible area of the retroperitoneum is the midline supramesocolic sector, which contains the suprarenal aorta and its branches. If you try to get to the suprarenal aorta directly from the front, you will have to transect the stomach and pancreas and then struggle through the dense connective tissue and nerve plexuses surrounding the aorta. The Mattox maneuver allows you to accomplish this exposure simply by lifting the left-sided abdominal viscera off the posterior abdominal wall and rolling them to the right.

Begin by mobilizing the lower descending colon, as in a left colectomy. Pull the left colon toward you, identify and incise the white line of Toldt, and rapidly mobilize the descending colon from below toward the splenic flexure. Continue your move upward along the same line, which extends lateral to the spleen.

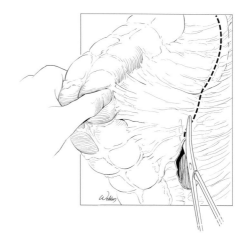

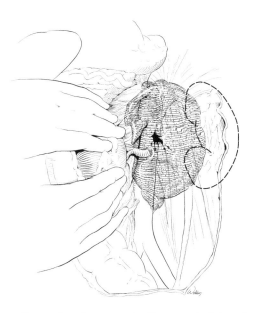

This move enables you to rotate the spleen, pancreas and left kidney in a medial direction toward the midline. As your hand sweeps from below upward and medially behind the left-sided organs, your plane is directly on the muscles of the posterior abdominal wall.

In most situations requiring this maneuver, the retroperitoneal hematoma will do much of the dissection for you. As it spreads laterally, the expanding hematoma lifts the left-sided viscera off the posterior abdominal wall, allowing you to perform the maneuver bluntly and rapidly.

> **An expanding central hematoma does the dissection for you**

You know you are in the correct plane as long as you can feel the posterior abdominal wall against your fingertips while you bluntly dissect behind the viscera with your hand. Continue the medial rotation all the way up to the diaphragmatic hiatus. You can then cut the left diaphragmatic crus laterally, and bluntly dissect around the aorta

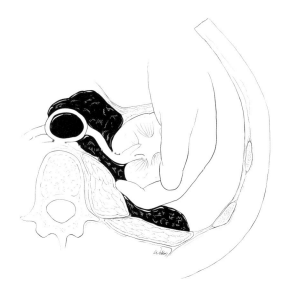

with your finger to gain access to the distal thoracic aorta as high as T6. This is a quick and easy way to gain proximal aortic control without opening the chest. The completed Mattox maneuver gives you access to the abdominal aorta as well as most of its branches, including the celiac, superior mesenteric, left renal and left iliac arteries.

If your target is the aorta itself or its anterior branches, rotate the left kidney with the other left-sided organs. If you leave the kidney in place by developing your plane anterior to it, you will restrict your access to the anterolateral aspect of the aorta. The left renal vein and artery will be in your way, and the left ureter will be vulnerable to injury. However, if your target is the left kidney or the renal vessels, leave the kidney in place.

Feel the muscles of the back against your fingertips

When you perform the Mattox maneuver for the first time, you discover (yet again) a discrepancy between neat illustrations and harsh reality. Don't say we didn't warn you. Once you have clamped the aorta proximally, it becomes a pulseless flaccid tube that is difficult to identify in a large retroperitoneal hematoma. To make matters worse, a thick layer of periaortic tissue separates the suprarenal aorta from your dissection plane, and you must divide it to gain the periaortic plane. We advise you to gain this plane at the infrarenal level, where it is much easier to identify, and then proceed up to the suprarenal aortic segment. In young hypotensive trauma patients, the aorta is constricted and considerably smaller than you expect.

It is not uncommon to injure the spleen during a rapid medial visceral rotation, so examine it closely when you have finished the maneuver. Another classic pitfall is avulsion of the left descending lumbar vein while mobilizing the left kidney. This treacherous vein comes off the left renal vein (LRV) and crosses over the left lateral aspect of the aorta immediately below the left renal artery. If you plan to work on the aorta around the level of the left renal vessels, it is a good idea to idenitify, ligate, and divide this lumbar vein to avoid avulsion during retraction of the mobilized left kidney.

Right-sided medial visceral rotation

Perform right-sided medial visceral rotation in three distinct stages. Each successive stage gives you progressively better exposure of the retroperitoneum.

The first stage is the classic Kocher maneuver, where you mobilize the duodenal loop and head of the pancreas. Identify the duodenum and incise the posterior peritoneum immediately lateral to it. Insinuate your hand behind the duodenum and head of the pancreas to begin lifting them up,

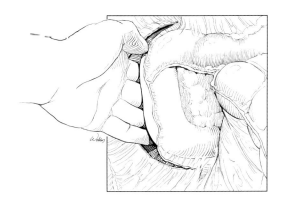

and continue mobilizing the duodenal loop from the common bile duct superiorly to the superior mesenteric vein (SMV) inferiorly. The hepatic flexure overlies the lower part of the duodenal loop, and you may have to mobilize it too. Now you can reflect the duodenal loop and head of the pancreas medially to see the IVC and the right renal hilum. Beware of injury to the right gonadal vein as it enters the IVC at this level.

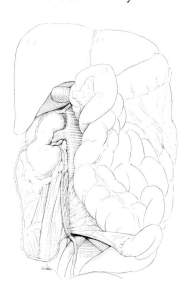

The second stage of a right-sided medial visceral rotation is the extended Kocher maneuver, which gives you wider exposure of the retroperitoneum. After completing the Kocher maneuver, carry the incision in the posterior peritoneum in a caudal direction toward the white line of Toldt, immediately lateral to the right colon. Note that this white line is in direct continuity with your previous incision around the duodenal loop. Fully mobilize the right colon and reflect it medially. The extended Kocher maneuver gives you access to the entire infrahepatic IVC, the right kidney and renal hilum, as well as the right iliac vessels.

Do a right-sided medial visceral rotation in three stages

The third stage is, you guessed it, a "super-extended Kocher maneuver," the widest possible exposure of the right-sided and midline retroperitoneal structures. This is the Cattell-Braasch maneuver. It is based on the anatomical observation that the small bowel mesentery is attached to the posterior abdominal wall along a short oblique line of fusion ("white line") that extends cranially and obliquely from the cecum to the ligament of Treitz.

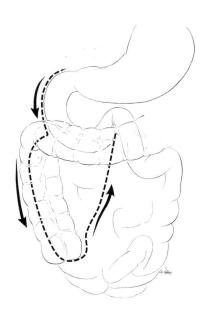

To perform the Cattell-Braasch maneuver, do an extended Kocher maneuver; then, carry the incision in the posterior peritoneum around the cecum. Now, gather the small bowel to the right and cranially, and incise the line of fusion of the small bowel mesentery to the posterior peritoneum from the medial side of the cecum to the ligament of Treitz, a surprisingly short distance. You should now be able to bring the small bowel and right colon out of the abdomen and swing them upward onto the anterior chest, a pretty remarkable sight.

The Cattell-Braasch maneuver begins at the common bile duct (CBD) and ends at the ligament of Treitz. When completed, it gives you a panoramic view of the entire inframesocolic retroperitoneum with access to the infrarenal aorta and IVC, as well as both renal arteries and veins and the iliac vessels on both sides. It also provides access to the third and fourth

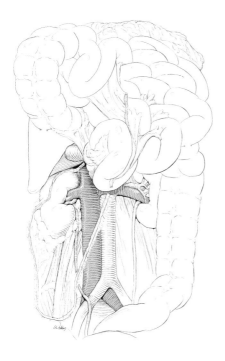

parts of the duodenum and the superior mesenteric vessels. It is an awesome exposure. We strongly recommend that you carefully study, understand, and memorize it because it is the key to approaching some of the most difficult abdominal injuries.

The major pitfall with right-sided medial visceral rotation is injury to the SMV at the root of the mesentery. Once you detach the right colon from its peritoneal attachment, it is hanging by its mesentery alone. An inadvertent pull will avulse the right colic vein off the SMV, resulting in unexpected bleeding from the root of the mesentery.

The Cattell-Braasch maneuver: from CBD to ligament of Treitz

Selecting an operative profile

Now it is time to decide which operative profile is appropriate for your patient: definitive repair or damage control (Chapter 1).

Injury Patterns Indicating the Need for Bail Out

Combined major vascular and hollow visceral injuries
Penetrating injury to the "surgical soul" (Chapter 8)
High-grade liver injury
Pelvic fracture with an expanding pelvic hematoma
Injuries requiring surgery in other cavities (chest, head, neck)

Temporary abdominal closure

How you close the abdomen after a damage control laparotomy depends on your personal preferences and institutional tradition. The specific technique is less important than providing effective containment of the swollen abdominal organs and protecting the exposed bowel.

Contain and protect the bowel with temporary abdominal closure

---

Our current preference is the vacuum pack. It is quick, easy and sutureless. It protects the bowel without abusing the fascia or skin and provides a means for collecting intra-abdominal fluid. Most importantly, it creates a physical barrier between the abdominal wall and the visceral mass. This barrier prevents adhesion formation between the bowel and the wall and extends the window of opportunity for early definitive abdominal closure.

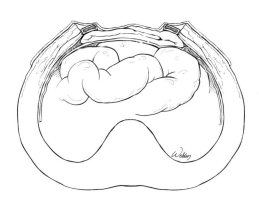

The vacuum pack is essentially a sandwich. The first layer is a wide polyethylene sheet that you spread over the abdominal viscera and carefully tuck between the bowel and the abdominal wall. Put two surgical towels over it, placed securely beneath the abdominal wall on all sides. This is the middle layer of the sandwich and its purpose is to absorb peritoneal fluid.

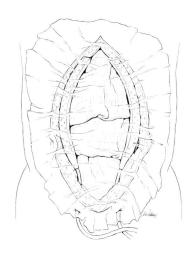

Now, place two silicone drains on the towels and bring them out through separate stab incisions. Cover the wound with a wide sterile polyester drape, completing the upper layer of the sandwich. Connect the suction tubing to a Y-connector, then to a suction source, and you're done.

Occasionally we still use a soft empty intravenous fluid bag for temporary abdominal closure. The bag is unfolded by cutting the seam and then sterilized. We suture it to the skin along the edge of the wound with a running heavy monofilament suture, preserving the fascia for the definitive closure. This technique is more time-consuming than the vacuum pack but provides inexpensive, atraumatic containment of the abdominal viscera.

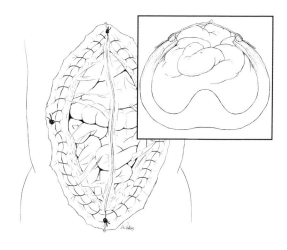

There isn't much we can tell you that you don't already know about definitive closure of a midline laparotomy incision. The correct technique is taking big bites close together, without tension. We do a mass closure (all layers) using a running heavy monofilament suture, beginning at both ends of the incision and working toward the middle. The cardinal sin is closure under tension. If you struggle to contain bulging or distended bowel, the patient will be much better off with temporary closure. Make a point of loosely approximating the fascia because this will accommodate subsequent swelling of the abdominal wall without causing fascial necrosis and dehiscence.

THE KEY POINTS

▶ Enter the belly with three sweeps of the knife and one educated finger.

▶ Stay away from old scars.

▶ Eviscerate the bowel early.

▶ In blunt trauma, begin with empirical packing.

▶ In penetrating trauma, eviscerate and go for the bleeder.

▶ Explore the supramesocolic and inframesocolic compartments.

▶ Keep retroperitoneal exploration targeted and limited.

▶ An expanding central hematoma does the dissection for you.

▶ Feel the muscles of the back against your fingertips.

▶ Do a right-sided medial visceral rotation in three stages.

▶ The Cattell-Braasch maneuver: from CBD to ligament of Treitz.

▶ Contain and protect the bowel with temporary abdominal closure.

Chapter 5
Fixing Tubes: The Hollow Organs

And if anything that I say should bear the appearance of arrogance or conceit, let me publicly confess that this book has arisen from a sorrowful contemplation of the many surgical errors which I have myself committed.

~ Harold Burrows, CBE
Pitfalls of Surgery, 2nd Edition,
London, Bailliere, Tindall and Cox, 1925

One of the most remarkable "corrective experiences" in surgical training comes during the morbidity and mortality conference, as you reluctantly rise to explain to an unsympathetic audience how you overlooked that bullet hole in the duodenum. From our own experience, no excuse sounds particularly convincing, so never get too complacent with the injured gut. It often hides some nasty traps.

Immediate concerns

Your first priorities are to control bleeding and contain spillage of intestinal content or urine. The bowel does not bleed much, but the mesentery does. If the bleeding vessel has retracted between the leaves of the mesentery, all you can see is an expanding mesenteric hematoma. Rather than waste time trying to identify the bleeder, simply apply pressure to the area. We usually use either the assistant's hand or long sponge-holding forceps applied

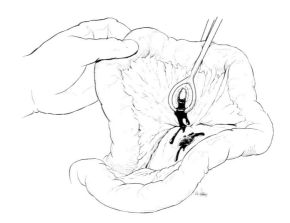

to the injured mesenteric segment, squeezing it gently between the ringed jaws.

When the bleeding laceration is close to the root of the mesentery, beware of a trap. Never jump in and blindly clamp or oversew the bleeder because you may destroy a superior mesenteric vessel or one of its major branches. A classic example is blunt avulsion of a proximal branch of the SMV, which can be the result of a deceleration injury or iatrogenic trauma from pulling hard on the mobilized right colon. You encounter brisk venous bleeding or a rapidly expanding hematoma at the base of the mesentery. Blind clamping may result in a transected and ligated SMV.

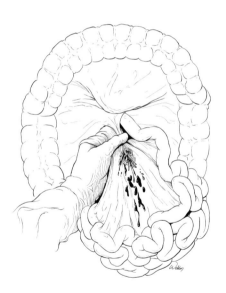

The correct approach is to insinuate your hand behind the mesentery and pinch the bleeding area between thumb and forefinger. This controls the bleeding. Now, carefully open the serosa, precisely define the injury, and fix it. With a blunt avulsion injury, you will have to fix a side-hole in the SMV.

Use soft bowel clamps to control spillage from stomach or bowel perforations. A hole in the stomach or bowel can also be temporarily whip-stitched with several big bites that will control mucosal bleeding. Pack a bladder perforation for temporary control.

Bleeding from the root of the mesentery is a trap

Missed injuries

Pay special attention to five locations where cursory inspection will often miss a hole in the gut:

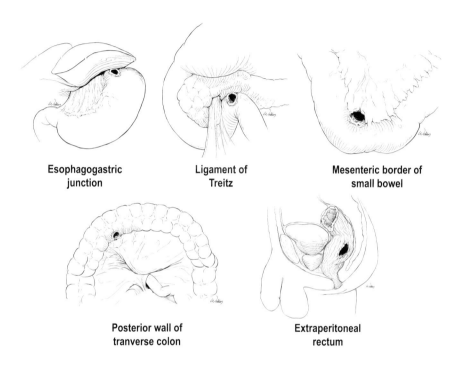

| Esophagogastric junction | Ligament of Treitz | Mesenteric border of small bowel |

| Posterior wall of tranverse colon | Extraperitoneal rectum |

Missing a gastric perforation has the most immediate consequences. Since the stomach is the most vascular organ of the gut, missing a hole means you will be back in the OR within a couple of hours facing a stomach the size of a watermelon filled with blood and clots. Much like a bleeding gastric ulcer, the most problematic and easily missed gastric injuries are located high on the lesser curve or in the posterior wall near the cardia. Mobilize the greater curve of the stomach by dividing the gastrocolic omentum. Open the lesser sac widely and lift the greater curve up to have a good look at the entire posterior wall.

In addition to a very meticulous exploration routine (Chapter 4), two safeguards help you to avoid missing a hidden injury to the GI tract:

1. Reconstruct the trajectory of the wounding agent. This trajectory must be linear and make sense. Bullets and knife blades do not disappear into thin air only to reappear out of nowhere in another part of the abdomen. You must be able to connect the dots. When the trajectory of the wounding missile is unclear or does not make sense, you probably are missing an injury.
2. Be concerned when finding an odd number of holes in the gut. Tangential wounds certainly occur, and occasionally a missile perforates only one wall, but this is uncommon. Therefore, an odd number of holes should prompt you to re-evaluate the area in search of a missed perforation. The only exception is a single stab wound to the anterior gastric wall, which is relatively common.

When examining the colon, it pays to be relentlessly paranoid. Because much of the colon is retroperitoneal or covered with omentum and pericolic fat, missing a small colonic perforation is easier than you think. Do not leave any subserosal hematoma on the colon, no matter how small and innocent-looking, without unroofing it by opening the overlying peritoneum. Very often, this seemingly innocent superficial staining hides a perforation. If the wounding agent passed close to the right or left colon, mobilize it and look carefully at the posterior wall.

The ureter, too, carries a high rate of missed injuries. Whenever a bullet trajectory passes anywhere near a ureter, mobilize the relevant side of the colon, identify the ureter, and trace it proximally and distally to ensure it is intact. Intravenous methylene blue dye helps identify a ureteral injury that is not immediately obvious.

Bullet trajectories are linear and must make sense

Choosing a repair technique

Now that you are ready to repair the injuries, choose an operative profile (Chapter 1) Are you going to do a definitive repair, or are you operating in damage control mode employing bail out solutions? While GI continuity is certainly desirable, the threat to the patient is contamination of the peritoneal cavity, a problem for which there is a range of almost instantaneous temporary solutions. You don't have to do a formal resection and reconstruction to prevent spillage.

Damage control for the bowel

The most expeditious way to prevent spillage from a perforation (and to achieve hemostasis at the same time) is to rapidly suture it using a single layer continuous stitch or, less commonly, a linear stapler. When operating in damage control mode, however, there are often multiple holes in several locations along the gut, and the patient's physiology and associated injuries do not allow you to patiently patch up hole after hole. You need a quick and effective spillage control solution. Here are the most commonly used options:

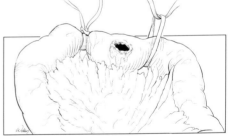

- Bowel interruption by stapling across with a linear stapler proximal and distal to the perforated segment, or ligating the bowel using a cotton tape without resection.

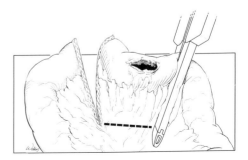

- Bowel resection without anastomosis is a good solution if the injury involves a bleeding mesentery. If you have to resect a considerable length of bowel in a patient *in extremis*, your quickest option is to sequentially fire a series of linear cutting staplers with vascular loads across the mesentery close to the bowel wall. If residual oozing from the stapler line persists, rapidly underrun it with a continuous monofilament stitch.

◆ Stapled partial gastric resection without reconstruction for a devastating gastric injury is a third option. This stapled emergency gastrectomy is a staged procedure - with resection during the initial bail out laparotomy and reconstruction at later reoperation.

During a bail out laparotomy, avoid external stomas, if possible. The abdominal wall swells up postoperatively, and the stoma often retracts or becomes ischemic. By creating a stoma you are also making definitive abdominal closure more difficult.

> **You can control spillage from the injured gut without resection**

Urological damage control

Urine spillage into the peritoneal cavity carries a much lower short-term risk of infection than intestinal spillage. If time is critical and you need to get out of the abdomen, tie off a transected ureter and plan a percutaneous nephrostomy if the patient survives. If you have no time to repair an injured bladder, just pack it and rely on a Foley catheter for drainage - a suboptimal but acceptable solution in extreme circumstances.

If you have a few minutes, intubate the injured or transected ureter proximally using any available thin catheter (such as a pediatric feeding tube). Secure the ureter to this drain with a tie and exteriorize the drain through the abdominal wall. Leave the distal ureter alone. It will not leak.

The biggest mistake you can make with a ureteral injury is to mobilize and dissect out the ureter in an attempt to better define the injury. You will only jeopardize the blood supply of the injured ureter and make subsequent reconstruction more difficult. If you are not going to repair it, just divert the urine and don't fiddle with the ureter.

Close a bladder injury with a quick running stitch. It doesn't have to be a multilayered formal repair if you are pressed for time; a single layer will do just fine. While always the best option, suture closure may not be feasible with a very large defect. On those rare occasions, you may elect to bail out by intubating both ureters and tightly packing the open bladder for hemostasis.

> **Drainage is an excellent damage control option for the ureter**

Definitive repair techniques

The stomach and distal esophagus

Repair gastric perforations using a suture or stapler. On rare occasions, massive destruction of the stomach requires a partial gastrectomy.

The cardia is the part of the stomach most difficult to visualize and repair, especially in obese patients. Approach these problematic injuries systematically. First, optimize your exposure. Is the incision extending as far up as possible? Is your retractor doing useful work? Should you insert an upper hand retractor? Is the patient tilted head up? Next, mobilize the EG junction as if you were going to do a vagotomy. We do realize this is rapidly becoming a lost art, but in this situation it is the key maneuver. Take down the left triangular ligament of the liver, fold up the left lateral lobe, open the posterior peritoneum overlying the esophagus along the "white line," and encircle the esophagus with your finger. This gives you good access to the injury.

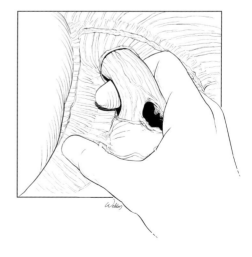

Sometimes you have to develop a creative technical solution for a proximal gastric injury. If you cannot roll the distal esophagus and cardia to expose the injury because it is posterior, open the anterior wall of the stomach longitudinally near the cardia, then identify and repair the high posterior perforation from within the stomach.

Injuries to the distal (abdominal) esophagus require the same mobilization of the EG junction and careful definition of the injury. If you are operating in damage control mode and there is no time for meticulous dissection and repair, insert a large suction drain into the open esophagus and bring it out through the abdominal wall, creating a controlled fistula. This effective temporary solution leaves the door open for later reconstruction.

We repair a simple laceration of the distal esophagus using a single layer suture after careful debridement of the perforation, and we always drain the area. You can use the cardia of the stomach as a serosal patch (Thal's patch) to buttress the repair. Very rarely, you will encounter a devastating injury that has destroyed the EG junction and requires resection of the distal esophagus and proximal stomach - a proximal gastrectomy. These patients typically have multiple associated injuries and need a rapid bail out solution. Transect the stomach across the body using a linear stapler, preserving as much distal stomach as possible. Lift the proximal part of the injured stomach and mobilize it along the lesser and greater curves all the way up to the esophagus. Divide the mobilized esophagus as low as possible and remove the destroyed part of the proximal stomach. Secure the open esophageal stump to the diaphragm to prevent retraction into the chest, and insert a closed suction drain into the lumen. This damage control solution leaves the patient with a stapled distal gastric remnant and a drained open esophageal stump.

Access proximal gastric injuries by mobilizing the EG junction

---

The small bowel

Before repairing a hole in the small bowel make sure the edges of the perforation are healthy and oozing nicely. If the bowel wall is bluish or traumatized, debride it. This is especially important with high-velocity gunshot wounds where tissue damage around the hole can be extensive. Common sense dictates repair of bowel perforations in a transverse orientation, rather than longitudinally, to avoid narrowing the lumen. Joining adjacent holes into a single laceration will save you time and trouble. Holes on the mesenteric border of the bowel can be tricky to fix. Carefully mobilize the adjacent mesentery to see the entire defect clearly before you begin sewing.

Expect some difficulty with injuries to the most proximal jejunal segment around the ligament of Treitz. The key is to mobilize the ligament and free the proximal jejunum. Rarely, you may have to do a complete Cattell-Braasch maneuver (Chapter 4) to get to the fourth portion of the duodenum and its transition into the proximal jejunum.

Repair the bowel using the technique you are most comfortable with. One of us prefers to use a single layer continuous stitch for most GI suture lines (including the stomach), while the other prefers a double layer technique. Both are safe if performed correctly, resulting in an inverted well-vascularized suture line without tension. If you must do a bowel resection, preserve bowel length and minimize the number of suture lines. The fewer suture lines you create, the better.

> **Preserve bowel length and keep suture lines to a minimum**

Colon and rectum

If you can close the colon laceration with a simple suture - just do it. No amount of peritoneal contamination should dissuade you from doing a straightforward primary repair. But what if the injured colonic segment must be resected?

For a right-sided or transverse colon injury, the answer is simple: do a right colectomy and join the terminal ileum to the transverse colon. This safe anastomosis is unlikely to cause you grief. The question becomes more interesting (and more controversial) in the left colon. Your options are to do a colocolostomy or to close the distal colon as a Hartman's pouch, bringing out the proximal segment as a colostomy. An extended right colectomy and ileocolostomy in the descending colon is a valid alternative, but it is seldom used in trauma because it is time-consuming.

In recent years, resecting and joining the unprepared left colon has become a fashionable option. Many surgeons talk about it; fewer do it, and some have had occasion to regret it. We belong to the latter group. Our preference for extensive left colon damage is resection and colostomy. We may occasionally do a colocolostomy for an isolated colon injury in a young stable patient who can tolerate a leak. We would not even contemplate it in a patient who has sustained massive physiological insult, is elderly and frail, or underwent other repairs that may leak. A case in point is the explosive combination of left colon and left kidney repairs, where a leak from one suture line puts the other repair in immediate jeopardy.

> **Many surgeons talk about colocolostomy for trauma; fewer do it**

Deal with an injury to the intraperitoneal rectum exactly as you would handle a perforated left colon. Management of trauma to the extraperitoneal rectum used to be an elaborate ritual that included total diversion, repair of the injury, washout of the distal rectal stump, and pre-sacral drainage. The current approach is much simpler:

1. Try to identify the injury using a rigid proctoscope. Repair it only if it is easily accessible. If you suspect a rectal injury but cannot prove it, perform an empirical fecal diversion. A temporary colostomy is a nuisance; a missed lower rectal injury can be fatal.
2. Do a sigmoid loop colostomy. When properly constructed at skin-level, it is totally diverting. Some surgeons use a linear stapler to close the colon immediately distal to the colostomy, or you can simply tie the sigmoid with a heavy polypropylene suture and anchor the stitch to the fascia.

3. Don't irrigate the rectal stump and don't insert a prosacral drain. Neither is necessary.

Divert the fecal stream away from extraperitoneal rectal injuries

---

Bladder and ureter injuries

Here, we can summarize our advice in a single word: DON'T! When possible, ask a urologist to perform definitive repair of an injured bladder or ureter. The urologist has a better grasp of the various technical options and how to choose the best one for a specific situation. Furthermore, the urologist will also manage any complications and undertake long-term follow-up. Whenever possible, we adhere to this principle even with straightforward intraperitoneal bladder injuries. If a urologist is not available, damage control is always a sound option.

THE KEY POINTS

▶   Bleeding from the root of the mesentery is a trap.

▶   Bullet trajectories are linear and must make sense.

▶   You can control spillage from the injured gut without resection.

▶   Drainage is an excellent damage control option for the ureter.

▶   Access proximal gastric injuries by mobilizing the EG junction.

▶   Preserve bowel length and keep suture lines to a minimum.

▶   Many surgeons talk about colocolostomy for trauma; fewer do it.

▶   Divert the fecal stream away from extraperitoneal rectal injuries.

Chapter 6
The Injured Liver: Ninja Master

*No battle plan survives the first five
minutes of contact with the enemy.*

~ Field Marshal Helmuth von Moltke

If trauma surgery is a contact sport, the badly injured liver is the Ninja Master: a vicious, cunning and lethal adversary. When you come face-to-face with a massively bleeding liver, glance at the OR clock and then at the anesthesiology team frantically pouring blood products into a rapid infusion device. You have a window of about 20 minutes and roughly 8-10 units of blood to stop the bleeding. That's all. Take much longer, lose more blood, or make an error in judgment or technique, and the Ninja Master wins again.

Obtain temporary control of bleeding

Once inside the abdomen, quickly look at the undersurface of the liver and swipe your hand over the superior hepatic surface on both sides of the falciform ligament. If there is a significant liver injury, you will see or feel it. At this point it is tempting to start fixing the injury - don't! An obvious liver injury is often just one of several sources of hemorrhage and not necessarily the most important one. Resist your natural tendency to zoom in on the bleeding liver as your prime target before rapidly assessing the rest of the abdomen.

Your first priority with a bleeding liver is to stop the bleeding. The three options for temporary control are manual compression, temporary packing, and the Pringle maneuver. Each option is useful for specific operative circumstances.

◆ Have your assistant reach across the operating table and *manually compress* the injured lobe between the palms of both hands, an excellent way to gain temporary control of a badly shattered lobe. It also allows you to begin hepatic mobilization around the compressing hands.

◆ *Temporary packing* is a good initial move, especially if you are not sure if the liver is the major source of bleeding. Rapidly compress the injured lobe in a sandwich of laparotomy packs placed above and below it (Chapter 2). You will return shortly for a closer look and definitive hemostasis.

◆ If the liver is bleeding despite temporary packing, consider *inflow occlusion* of the portal triad, the well-known Pringle maneuver. Poke a hole in an avascular portion of the lesser omentum to the left of the portal triad, insert an educated finger into the lesser sac, and gently pinch the portal triad between thumb and forefinger. If the maneuver is working and bleeding stops, replace your fingers with a large 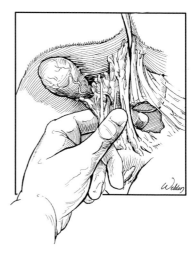 aortic vascular clamp, a Rummel tourniquet, or (if none of these is immediately available) a soft non-crushing bowel clamp. Note the time. Nobody knows for sure how long the portal triad of a trauma patient can remain clamped before ischemic damage occurs, but you have at least 30-45 minutes, probably more. Remove the clamp as quickly as you can.

Sometimes your temporary hemostatic maneuver fails and the bleeding continues. Barring a technical error (such as ineffective packing or an incorrectly performed Pringle maneuver), there are three possible reasons for ongoing hemorrhage:

◆ Packs do not control arterial bleeding. You need inflow occlusion.
◆ If the bleeding from the liver looks arterial despite inflow occlusion, the hepatic artery may have an anomalous origin. Try supraceliac aortic clamping.
◆ If dark blood is gushing from the deep recesses behind the liver, you are dealing with a retrohepatic venous injury. If you aren't sure, ask the anesthesiologist to momentarily disconnect the patient from the ventilator. If the bleeding abates, your suspicion is confirmed and you and your patient are in deep trouble. Incise the falciform ligament, grab it with a clamp, and push gently posteriorly and to the left. This tilts the liver backward and may temporarily control the bleeding while you consider your options and organize your attack.

Control the liver temporarily using hand, pack, or clamp

Mobilize the injured lobe

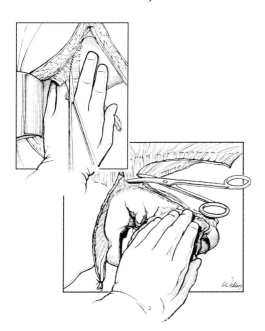

Unless the hepatic laceration is peripheral and anterior, you cannot assess or repair it until you have delivered the injured lobe to the midline, much like the injured spleen. To mobilize the left lobe, divide the falciform ligament between clamps and then release it all the way up to the diaphragm, exposing the areolar tissue of the bare area of the liver. Then divide the left triangular ligament and continue the incision into the anterior and posterior coronary ligaments. Beware of the phrenic vein that is very close to your scissors.

Similarly, putting your hand behind the right lobe and rotating it medially stretches the right triangular ligament and allows you to divide it safely. Continue the mobilization by releasing the anterior coronary ligament (taking care not to injure the liver capsule or the right diaphragm) and then the posterior coronary ligament. Your goal is to deliver the entire right lobe to the midline.

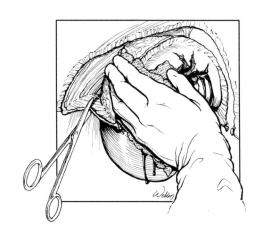

Be liberal with your mobilization, but also be careful; the hepatic veins and IVC are waiting for a careless move, and the small accessory veins entering the IVC below the right hepatic vein are easily avulsed with a careless move.

Mobilize the injured lobe to deal with it face-to-face

Here, a deadly pitfall awaits you. Massive gushes of dark blood coming through a deep laceration in the liver or from behind it likely represent an injury to the retrohepatic veins. Mobilizing the liver in this situation is a recipe for disaster. You will lose containment, and the patient will exsanguinate from uncontrolled venous hemorrhage before you even realize your mistake. So, if you have any suspicion of a retrohepatic venous injury, don't mobilize the liver.

Small problem or BIG TROUBLE?

Nowhere is the distinction between small problems and BIG TROUBLE (Chapter 2) more useful than in hepatic trauma. Small problems are liver injuries that you can fix with a direct, simple maneuver: the diathermy, a liver stitch, or a local hemostatic agent. The injury is accessible and blood loss is not dramatic. Most liver injuries belong in this category.

BIG TROUBLE is a high-grade injury with massive blood loss, and you are in imminent danger of losing your patient. The decision whether the injury is a small problem or BIG TROUBLE is the key strategic decision in hepatic trauma.

Deal with low-grade injuries directly. If a superficial laceration is not bleeding, leave it alone. If there is slow oozing, direct pressure for a few minutes often stops the bleeding. Your hemostatic efforts should be proportional to the magnitude of the injury (Chapter 2).

With deeper lacerations, have your assistant pinch the edges of the laceration, turn the cautery to KILL, and blast the raw bleeding surface, focusing on the disrupted edges of the hepatic capsule. Apply the cautery to a metal sucker tip to achieve a wider effect. Use an Argon Beam Coagulator, if available, to thoroughly barbeque the raw surface. Use a topical hemostatic agent you are familiar with from elective surgery.

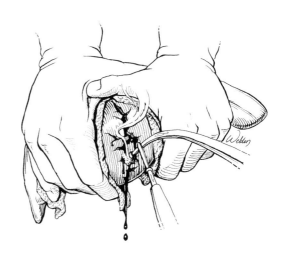

Next, consider hepatorrhaphy. For your sutures to hold, you need a reasonably intact capsule and a more or less linear laceration that can be approximated side-to-side. We typically suture hepatic lacerations with 0 chromic on a blunt-tip large needle, creating a row of horizontal mattress sutures. The chromic suture slides through the hepatic parenchyma, and the large curved needle enables you to obtain a good bite of tissue.

With BIG TROUBLE, you are operating in damage control mode. The key to success is your ability to stop the operation and organize your attack on the injury, rather than get carried away and attempt heroic maneuvers on an exsanguinating patient (Chapter 2). The rest of this chapter describes the techniques we have found most useful in battles with hepatic BIG TROUBLE.

> **Decide if you are dealing with a small problem or BIG TROUBLE**

"Packing plus"

Packing is the technique you will use most commonly for a high-grade liver injury. If you have packed the liver early as a temporary hemostatic maneuver and the bleeding has stopped, you have achieved hemostasis. Removing packs at this point is a mistake.

When you cannot be sure that you have complete hemostasis with packing, especially if you had to remove the packs for bleeding but did not find any discrete arterial bleeders, consider *packing plus* - immediate postoperative angiography with selective embolization as a hemostatic adjunct. This is a risky undertaking in a critical patient and involves mobilizing resources that may not be available to you. However, if it is a realistic option at your institution, selective embolization of arterial bleeders deep within the liver can be lifesaving. If your OR has intraoperative angiographic capabilities, the decision is easy, and embolization is possible without moving the patient. It is crucial to make the decision early. Decide that you are going for angiography while you are repacking the liver, not three hours later.

Keep in mind that angiographic embolization is an *adjunct* to effective packing, not a substitute for sloppy hemostasis. If you didn't pack the liver properly, angiographic embolization will not save your patient.

> **Consider angiographic embolization as an adjunct to packing**

Deep liver sutures

Deep liver sutures have a bad reputation. They cause necrosis of tissue incorporated in the stitch, predisposing to infection or "liver fever" from necrosis without infection. Don't let this bad reputation rob you of an effective weapon in your battle with the Ninja Master, especially if you don't have much experience with the injured liver or need a rapid bail out solution. A live patient with some hepatic necrosis is far better than a dead one.

When placing deep liver sutures, you must have an intact capsule to hold them. When tying, tighten very carefully, as if you are tying a suture through refrigerated butter. Look for blanching of the liver parenchyma beneath the suture, which signifies the suture is tight. Choose a suture configuration that is best for the specific anatomic circumstances: horizontal (or sometimes vertical) mattress, a figure of 8, or a simple through-and-through, with or without an omental buttress. Regardless of your chosen configuration, to obtain a good purchase of hepatic tissue, the needle must always move perpendicular to the surface of the liver and not obliquely.

A trap with deep liver sutures is early postoperative bleeding. As the injured liver swells, the sutures may cut through the edematous parenchyma with loss of the hemostatic effect and rebleeding.

Deep liver sutures are not a crime

Hepatotomy with selective vascular ligation

This is a useful technique to control bleeding from deep in the liver, especially if you are an experienced surgeon. When you see arterial hemorrhage coming from a deep laceration, rather than trying to close a deep laceration, *open it wider* and go in hot pursuit of the hidden arterial bleeders. In other words, go to the heart of danger to find safety.

With a Pringle maneuver in place, incise the hepatic capsule with the cautery to extend the laceration. Then, open the parenchyma in the direction of the injury using finger fracture (or a blunt metal instrument). As you go deeper into the liver, gently insert a pair of narrow Deaver retractors into the laceration to facilitate exposure. Using this technique, the liver parenchyma disintegrates between your fingers while the ductal structures remain intact and can be controlled (with ligatures, sutures or metal hemostatic clips) and divided, enabling you

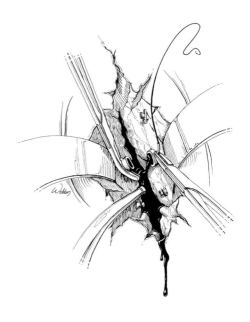

to widen the gap and go deeper. We prefer to suture-ligate all significant bleeders because suture-ligatures do not slip when you continue working in the area. If you use metal hemostatic clips, apply two clips to each ductal structure (double clipping) to prevent slipping. Occasionally, an injured large intralobar vein will require lateral repair using 5:0 polypropylene.

Hepatotomy with selective vascular ligation is a neat concept, but its application in the real world is less straightforward than the preceding description leads you to believe. It involves significant ongoing blood loss, is time-consuming, and may result in iatrogenic injury to a major hepatic duct or hilar vessel. Use it only after you have organized your attack and when the patient is resuscitated and can tolerate additional blood loss. If you don't have much experience with hepatic trauma, deep liver sutures can be a simpler alternative.

Hepatotomy with selective ligation is easier said than done

The viable omental pedicle

On completion of finger fracture hepatotomy and selective vascular ligation, you are left with a considerable dead space. Filling it with omentum is a good idea. The same applies to a deep liver suture, where a pack of omentum can help you achieve hemostasis. In fact, when dealing with the injured liver, the greater omentum is one of your best friends.

If you have time, mobilize the greater omentum off the transverse colon along the bloodless line. Select a healthy chunk, typically from the right side, and separate it by dividing the omentum longitudinally toward the greater curve of the stomach. Swing the mobilized tongue of omentum up into the injured liver, and fix it to the liver capsule with several loose stitches. Another option is stuffing the omental tongue tightly into the laceration, filling the space, and then approximating the laceration loosely with several liver stitches over the omental pack. Some surgeons use omentum for packing from within instead of laparotomy pads or gauze rolls.

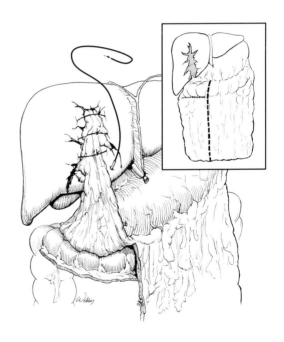

Fill large parenchymal defects with omentum

Balloon tamponade

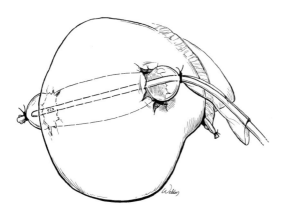

When dealing with a through-and-through (transfixing) liver injury, which may occasionally involve both lobes, remember the option of balloon tamponade - an ingenious and easy solution to a very bad problem. The alternative is extensive tractotomy to achieve direct hemostasis.

If the tract is wide (2cm in diameter or more), we use a Blakemore tube. Insert the tube into the tract so that the gastric balloon, inflated outside the exit wound from the liver, will serve as an anchor to prevent dislodgement of the tube. Then, gently inflate the esophageal balloon in the tract until bleeding stops.

If the tract is too narrow or too short for a Blakemore tube, we improvise a balloon from a red rubber catheter and a Penrose drain. Tie off one end of the drain with two heavy silk ties. Tie the other end around the catheter, creating a sausage-shaped balloon. Check the balloon for leaks by injecting saline through the red rubber catheter and clamping it. If the device is working, insert the balloon into the tract and bring the other end of the catheter out through a stab incision in the abdominal wall, as if it were a drain. Inflate the balloon and watch bleeding stop as if by magic. Secure the red rubber catheter to the skin and make sure the end is clamped.

You can safely begin removing the balloon at the bedside after 24-48 hours. First deflate the device, but keep it in place for 6-8 hours. If there is no clinical evidence of bleeding, pull the balloon out like you would any other drain.

Balloon tamponade is a cool solution for a bad problem

Resectional debridement

When a substantial part of the hepatic lobe is destroyed and bleeding profusely, the most expedient option is resectional debridement. Have your assistant manually compress the non-injured liver parenchyma around the area you wish to resect. If the lobe is properly mobilized, often your assistant will be able to completely encircle the injured part, minimizing blood loss while you do the resection.

Turn the cautery to maximum and use it to define a line of resection that is immediately outside the injured area in healthy hepatic tissue. Always resect immediately outside the injured area where the vessels are intact and have not retracted; never resect within injured tissue. This is the key maneuver of resectional debridement.

Perform finger fracture (the "pinched corn bread" maneuver) and selective ligation along your chosen line of resection. The simplest example for use of this technique is resection of the left lateral lobe along a line immediately to the left of the falciform ligament. Some surgeons use a linear cutting stapler with a vascular staple load to facilitate this non-anatomic hepatic resection.

Much like hepatotomy and selective vascular ligation, resectional debridement takes time and involves considerable blood loss. Don't attempt it in a patient rapidly dying on the operating table. Organize your attack and resuscitate the patient before you begin.

Perform resectional debridement in healthy liver tissue

Other techniques

The trauma literature is replete with many techniques that resourceful surgeons have developed for dealing with bad liver injuries. One example is the absorbable mesh wrap. By snugly fitting a "pita" of absorbable mesh around a shattered lobe, the advocates of this technique achieve effective tamponade, avoiding the need for packing. We find this technique cumbersome and do not use it.

Hepatic artery ligation is still mentioned in trauma texts as an effective hemostatic technique. Some surgeons use it for ongoing arterial bleeding not controlled by other means. We have not used this technique in years.

How about draining the injured liver? This is a somewhat controversial topic. One of us routinely drains all high-grade liver injuries using a closed suction drain, while the other almost never does.

Retrohepatic venous injury

Gushing dark blood from a deep hole in the liver or from behind and around it usually means an injury to either the retrohepatic IVC or hepatic veins. These encounters are rare, brief, and brutal. More often than not, the result is on-table exsanguination and a very frustrated surgeon.

The retrohepatic veins are the least accessible vascular structures in the abdomen. You cannot get to them and define the injury unless you somehow control the hemorrhage. The classic technique to accomplish this is the atriocaval (Schrock) shunt, one of the "great technical feats" of trauma surgery. You will find elegant illustrations depicting the technique in every major trauma book, but not in this one. Why? Because in real life it very rarely works. In fact, even in the most experienced hands, the atriocaval shunt has dismal results.

Instead of engaging in futile heroics, use common sense. The retrohepatic veins are a low-pressure system amenable to containment and tamponade. Your best move, therefore, is to contain the injury, not try and fix it. A retrohepatic venous injury bleeds freely only if one or more of its containment structures is disrupted. These structures are the suspensory ligaments of the liver (marking the borders of the bare area), the right diaphragm, and the liver itself.

Your realistic options for dealing with a retrohepatic venous injury are:

◆   Leave a contained retrohepatic hematoma alone. Don't mobilize the liver and don't try to explore the hematoma. Just move on to other injuries (and count your blessings).

◆ If dark blood is gushing out from a deep hole in the liver paronchyma, plug the hole. Pack it with a laparotomy pad, viable omentum, or balloon tamponade. Whatever it takes - just plug the hole.

◆ Don't open "Pandora's Box" (Chapter 10). A hole in the right diaphragm bleeding into the chest in a patient with penetrating thoracoabdominal trauma can hide a retrohepatic venous injury. Simply close the hole and don't mobilize the liver.

◆ When bleeding emanates from behind the liver, try to determine if the source is below or behind the liver. Injuries to the IVC below the liver (the pararenal and suprarenal segments) are accessible to direct repair. It's difficult, but can be done.

◆ If the suspensory ligaments of the liver are disrupted, your best chance to control the bleeding is packing the area quickly and tightly. With limited disruption of the ligaments, you may be able to re-establish containment with packing. With massive disruption, often associated with a high-grade liver injury, the battle is usually lost even before you start packing.

Should you even consider an atriocaval shunt? It may be a realistic option, but only under very specific circumstances. You need two teams of experienced surgeons who can work simultaneously in the abdomen and chest, the necessary equipment must be available, and bleeding must be temporarily controlled while the effort is organized.

The technique entails a median sternotomy, a purse-string suture in the right atrial appendage using 3:0 polypropylene and a Rummel tourniquet, and encircling the supradiaphragmatic IVC inside the pericardium with an umbilical tape on another Rummel tourniquet. We use a size 9 endotracheal tube, clamped proximally, with a side-hole cut 17cm from the tip. We insert the shunt with the curve of the tube facing anteriorly so that the tip does not end up in the hepatic veins. The surgeon operating in the abdomen directs placement to prevent shunt extrusion through the injury. The balloon on the tube obviates the need for encircling the suprarenal IVC in the abdomen. The shunt does not provide a completely dry field but does allow you to see the injury and get to it.

In retrohepatic venous injury, restore containment - don't be a hero

The "evil green eye"

For obvious reasons, injuries to the biliary tract are often associated with hepatic trauma, and leaking bile is a lower priority than spurting blood. What are your damage control and definitive repair options for the injured biliary tract?

A perforated gallbladder can be repaired, drained, or removed. The definitive solution is that rare, almost extinct operation - open cholecystectomy. In a crashing coagulopathic patient, taking the gallbladder off the liver is not the smartest move in the book. Instead, either repair the laceration with a single layer of absorbable suture or drain the gallbladder with a cholecystostomy tube inserted through the injured fundus and secured with a purse-string suture.

The damage control solution for common bile duct injuries is external drainage. If you need to bail out in a hurry, cannulate the proximal duct and bring the drain out through the abdominal wall. Ligating or clipping the common duct of a patient in dire straights is an acceptable damage control option, but will require a complex reconstructive solution at reoperation. If you can't see the leaking hole, a drain in Morrison's pouch is good enough. The leak can be managed later by ERCP and endoscopic stenting.

If you can clearly see the injury and the common bile duct is wide enough to accommodate a T-tube, this is a good bail out option. However, the common bile duct of most young trauma patients is narrow and delicate, and inserting a T-tube into it may well buy your patient a postoperative stricture.

The definitive repair of extrahepatic biliary injuries depends on the magnitude of damage. Repair a simple laceration (partial transection) with an absorbable suture and an external drain. Although it is not mandatory, we insert a T-tube in the common bile duct if it is of sufficient caliber to accommodate at least an 8 French tube. If you decide to use a T-tube, always insert it through a separate choledochotomy rather than through the injury site to prevent a stricture.

Definitive repair of complete or near-complete transection of the bile duct is with a Roux-en-Y hepaticojejunostomy. Before you begin, a cholecystectomy will facilitate access and exposure of the injured duct.

Drainage is the bail out solution for biliary trauma

THE KEY POINTS

▶ Control the liver temporarily using hand, pack, or clamp.

▶ Mobilize the injured lobe to deal with it face-to-face.

▶ Decide if you are dealing with a small problem or **BIG TROUBLE**.

▶ Consider angiographic embolization as an adjunct to packing.

▶ Deep liver sutures are not a crime.

▶ Hepatotomy with selective ligation is easier said than done.

▶ Fill large parenchymal defects with omentum.

▶ Balloon tamponade is a cool solution for a bad problem.

▶ Perform resectional debridement in healthy liver tissue.

▶ In retrohepatic venous injury, restore containment - don't be a hero.

▶ Drainage is the bail out solution for biliary trauma.

Chapter 7
The "Take-outable" Solid Organs

*For every complex problem, there is a
solution that is simple, neat, and wrong.*

~ H.L. Mencken

Although they belong to different organ systems, the spleen, kidney, and distal pancreas have a lot in common. From the trauma surgeon's perspective, they are close relatives because they are "take-outable."

Consider the fundamental difference between an injured spleen and a bleeding liver. The spleen has a single accessible vascular pedicle that you can rapidly get to and control. The liver has two vascular pedicles (one in the hepatoduodenal ligament and the other behind the liver where the hepatic veins drain into the IVC), only one of which is easily accessible. Total vascular control of the liver is, therefore, tricky business. It is not a take-outable organ in the bleeding trauma patient.

It never made sense to us to consider both head and distal pancreas (body and tail) in the same chapter. From the trauma surgeon's point of view they are different organs. The distal pancreas can be easily resected, while the pancreatic head requires a very big whack.

The spleen, kidney, and distal pancreas are take-outable abdominal solid organs. They can bleed a lot before you get to them, but once you have gained control of the vascular pedicle, bleeding stops immediately. The key to vascular control is mobilizing each organ and lifting it toward the midline. In stark contrast, resection of a "non-take-outable" solid organ such as the liver or the head of the pancreas is a prohibitive technical undertaking in the trauma patient unless the injury has done most of the resection for you.

At first glance, bringing together three solid organs from three different organ systems under the same roof may seem strange to you. Bear with us, and your understanding and comfort level in dealing with these injuries will grow.

| **The spleen, kidney, and tail of the pancreas are take-outable** |

The spleen

Mobilization

If you see or suspect a splenic injury, your first move must be mobilizing the spleen to the midline. You can neither adequately assess nor repair the spleen without having it in your hand. Mobilizing the spleen is the key maneuver that unlocks the left upper quadrant. It brings the spleen and distal pancreas out of the dark recesses of the abdomen into your incision and exposes the left kidney. While mobilizing the spleen is a basic maneuver in surgery, performing it quickly, blindly, and in a pool of blood is not as it appears in the illustrations.

| **Mobilize the spleen to unlock the left upper quadrant** |

You may not have heard this before, but in reality (as opposed to the virtual world of the surgical atlas), there are two kinds of spleens: mobile and stuck.

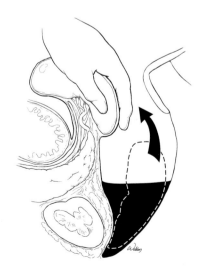

The mobile spleen has lax spleno-renal and splenophrenic ligaments and no adhesions to the abdominal wall. By putting your non-dominant hand over the splenic convexity and pulling medially, you can bring the mobile spleen toward you, almost to the midline. You still have to cut the splenorenal ligament behind the spleen, but this is easy because you do it almost in the midline rather than high up in the left upper abdomen.

The stuck spleen is, you guessed it, stuck. To get it to the midline, you have to deal with two obstacles. The first are adhesions between the splenic capsule and the abdominal wall that will not let you pass your hand over the splenic convexity. If there is little or no bleeding, you can take your time and sharply divide the adhesions with scissors or cautery. But if you are working in a pool of blood, just do whatever it takes to quickly get them out of the way with your fingers, scissors, or both. Damage to the splenic capsule doesn't matter since the spleen is coming out anyway.

The second obstacle with the stuck spleen is a short and unyielding splenorenal ligament. Put your non-dominant hand over the spleen so the tips of your fingers rest on the membrane behind and lateral to it. This is the splenorenal ligament. Gently pull the spleen toward you to stretch the ligament. Working in a pool of blood, you often cannot see it, but you can easily *feel* it. Immediately beyond the tips of your fingers, make a nick in the stretched ligament with your scissors.

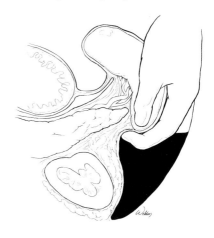

Enlarge the nick sharply (with scissors) or bluntly (with your fingers) up and around the spleen. Both the splenorenal and splenophrenic ligaments

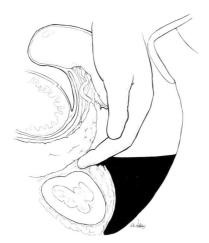

are avascular, and dividing them allows you to bring the spleen to the midline.

Palpate the left kidney and bluntly develop the plane behind the spleen and in front of the kidney, bringing the spleen and tail of the pancreas up into the wound. The pitfall here, especially in the presence of massive bleeding, is going behind the left kidney and discovering that you have brought it to the midline with you.

Once the spleen is mobilized and in your hand, bleeding control is not a problem. Pinch the splenic vascular pedicle, which includes both the gastrosplenic ligament (carrying the short gastric vessels) in front and the splenic hilum behind. Alternatively, place a soft bowel clamp or a large vascular clamp globally across the entire pedicle if you have other urgent business to attend to first. Think of it as the "Pringle maneuver of the spleen."

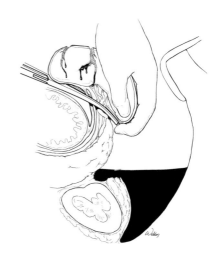

Rarely, on a particularly bad night, you may find yourself gazing in disbelief at the ruptured spleen from hell, a diseased organ so enlarged and stuck to the abdominal wall and diaphragm that rapidly developing a plane behind it is simply out of the question. In this case, your only option is to attack the spleen from the front. One quick way to control the splenic artery is to enter the lesser sac through the gastrocolic omentum and isolate the artery along the upper border of the pancreas. Another option is to go straight at the hilum. Gently pull the stomach toward you to put the gastrosplenic ligament on tension and divide it between clamps. Immediately behind it you will find the splenic hilar vessels. Clamp them and only then start your dissection to free and mobilize the devascularized spleen.

> ### Do what it takes to bring the spleen to the midline

Remove or repair?

You are now facing the key strategic decision in splenic trauma: remove or repair? Splenectomy or splenorrhaphy?

Your answers to the following four questions guide your decision.

1. What is the patient's trauma burden? Ongoing shock, severe associated injuries in or outside the abdomen - all are indications to rapidly put the spleen in a bucket.
2. What is the patient's age? Splenic preservation is much more important in kids. Splenorrhaphy also works better in the pediatric spleen because it has a thick capsule that holds sutures well.
3. How bad is the injury? Is a repair likely to work? Is there a hilar injury that makes repair much more difficult? Will a repair entail additional blood loss? Never make this decision with the spleen *in situ*. Always bring it to the midline and assess the injury with the spleen in your hand.
4. What is your experience with splenic repair? Have you done it before or is it a "read one, do one" situation? Is the injury amenable to a repair technique that you are comfortable with?

For splenic repair, consider trauma burden, age, injury, and experience

---

Completing the splenectomy

Contrary to the impression you may have from reading the trauma literature of the past decade, splenectomy is not a crime. It is often the safest and most expedient solution. One very effective technique of splenic preservation is the formalin jar.

Once you have the mobilized spleen in your hand, completing the splenectomy is easy. Clamp and divide the vessels of the splenic hilum from the back or side, whichever is most convenient. The key technical principle here is to stay very close to the spleen so you will not injure the tail of the pancreas or the stomach. For the sake of speed,

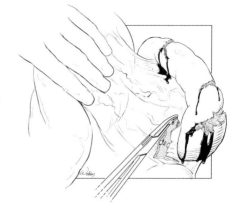

clamp only the proximal side of the line of resection. Clamping the spleen side wastes time since it comes out in a moment anyway. Serially clamp and divide the gastrosplenic ligament, taking care to stay away from the greater curve of the stomach. The splenocolic ligament is the only remaining attachment. Clamp and divide it, and the spleen is out.

Now pick up the clamps one-by-one, and ligate the vessels they are controlling. You may decide to doubly ligate or suture-ligate the hilar vessels. Re-examine the greater curve of the stomach to ensure you did not accidentally pinch the gastric wall. Much has been written about iatrogenic injury to the tail of the pancreas during splenectomy. This concern is much overrated. If you think that you may have injured the pancreas while removing the spleen, leave a closed suction drain in the splenic bed.

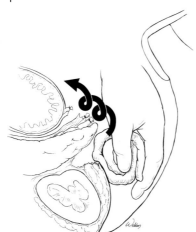

Lastly, check for hemostasis. Suck out all the blood and clots in the splenic fossa. Take a tightly rolled laparotomy pad, go to the deepest part of the splenic fossa, and slowly roll the pack toward you medially, over the area of the pancreatic tail and the greater curve. If you identify a bleeder, stop rolling and deal with it.

Stay close to the spleen

Fixing the injured spleen

If you decided to repair the spleen, use the simplest technical solution that will work. Choose from a limited menu of repair techniques that have worked for you in the past. Few surgeons have experience with a vast array of splenic repair methods. What are your realistic options?

Local pressure (with your hand or a pack), works in superficial lacerations and capsular avulsions. Your favorite local hemostatic agent can also help. The Argon beam coagulator, if available, does wonders for a larger raw surface or a deeper laceration.

Because the capsule of the adult spleen does not hold sutures well, use a monofilament suture that slides through the tissue, along with some kind of bolster or support. Our preferred technique is running a monofilament suture on a straight needle between two strips of Teflon on both sides of the laceration. Some surgeons use omentum as a bolster.

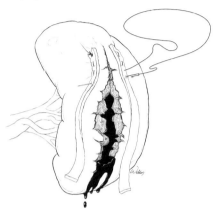

A severely injured or devitalized splenic pole may require a limited resection. Have your assistant manually compress the spleen just beyond the planned line of resection to control bleeding. Intermittently releasing the pressure shows you where the bleeders are so you can suture-ligate them or blast them with the Argon beam. You can then oversew the open splenic "stump" with mattress sutures between two strips of Teflon. If the spleen is flat rather than bulky, another option is using a linear stapler with 4.8mm staples. Bring the stapler to the line of transection and slowly close it so as not to break the capsule. Fire the stapler and amputate the splenic tissue distal to the stapled line.

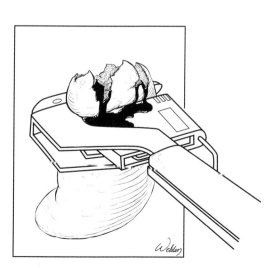

Don't persist if your repair doesn't work, and don't rely on the patient's clotting mechanism to stop ongoing oozing. "If it ain't dry, it's not working!" In an adult patient, we proceed with splenectomy if the first attempted repair fails. If you strongly believe that repair is still the best option for the patient, you may try a second time. A third attempt is playing with fire.

We have given you the limited menu of splenic repair techniques we use in our practice; sorry if you are disappointed. We have little experience with formal hemisplenectomy or the absorbable mesh wrap. We consider them unnecessarily risky acrobatics. In situations where these techniques would be required, we prefer to err on the side of caution and do a splenectomy.

Don't persist if splenorrhaphy doesn't work

The distal pancreas

Exploration

You can have a quick "rule out" look at the body and tail of the pancreas through the lesser sac by poking a hole in the gastrocolic omentum on the left (Chapter 4). However, if you see or suspect an injury, you need a wide exposure. Have your assistant pull the stomach upward and the transverse colon downward, and detach the greater omentum from the transverse colon along the bloodless line to open the full width of the lesser sac. With any sign of injury,

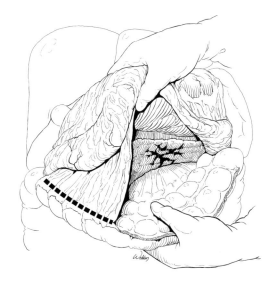

open the posterior peritoneum overlying the injured area. What you presume to be an innocent-looking minor hematoma or superficial laceration will often prove a serious injury when you unroof it and look it in the face.

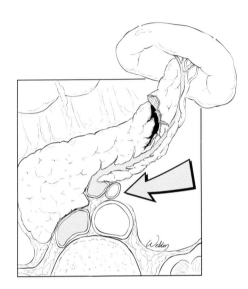

For significant injury, and especially if you are going to resect the distal pancreas, the quickest way to bring the body and tail into full view (including the posterior aspect of the gland) is to mobilize it out of its bed. Mobilize the spleen and continue to develop the plane behind the pancreatic tail and body until it can be lifted medially into the operative incision. Distal pancreatectomy without splenectomy is an elaborate exercise suitable mostly to an elective situation. We do not recommend nor use it in trauma patients.

Look at the pancreas from the front - but mobilize it from the left

---

Decision

Is there a ductal injury? This is the key question when assessing the injured pancreas. Sometimes you immediately see that the pancreas is transected or you can identify the injured duct in a deep wound. More often, you cannot rule out a ductal injury based on inspection and palpation alone. What then?

In a stable patient with no other major injuries, you can try a frustrating exercise called intraoperative pancreatography. Inject 20ml of contrast into the gallbladder through a needle and catheter and pray that it fills the pancreatic duct in a retrograde fashion through the ampulla. Proponents of this technique claim it works about half the time. In our experience it rarely does. Because they are totally unnecessary, we don't recommend other options like amputating the tail of the pancreas to find the duct or the absurd notion of making a duodenotomy to cannulate the papilla.

We prefer the common sense, expedient approach. If exploration reveals a deep injury likely to involve the duct, do not hesitate to perform a distal pancreatectomy, even without definitive proof of ductal injury. If we have a low suspicion or need to bail out quickly, we leave a drain adjacent to the injury and perform an ERCP as soon as possible after the operation, realizing that we may occasionally have to go back for a distal pancreatectomy.

You don't need photographs to deal with a pancreatic injury

Hemostasis and drainage

The damage control solution for injuries to the pancreatic body and tail is hemostasis and drainage. Pack the lesser sac for hemostasis. A drain converts the injury from a potential uncontrolled pancreatic leak into a controlled fistula that has a benign course and can be addressed later.

Definitive management of most distal pancreatic injuries is not much different than the damage control option. Stop bleeding from superficial lacerations and contusions using local hemostatic means. Don't suture the capsule of the pancreas because this is asking for trouble. Leave a large suction drain (or two) adjacent to the injury, feed the patient as early as possible, and remove the drain when it stops working. For pancreatic injuries that don't involve the duct, this is all you need to do.

When there is obvious ductal injury or when you have a strong suspicion about the duct but cannot prove it, do a distal pancreatectomy.

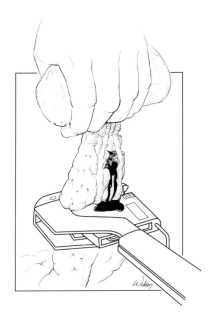

If you happen to come across the pancreatic duct, ligate it. Otherwise, don't spend time looking for it. Lift the spleen and the pancreas to the midline, take a linear stapler, place it across the body of the pancreas including the splenic vessels, and shoot. Amputate the distal pancreas and spleen and give the pancreatic stump a close look. Control any bleeding from the splenic vessels with a hemostatic stitch. One of us usually underruns the stapled line with a 3:0 monofilament non-absorbable suture; the other never does. Don't forget to leave a closed suction drain in the pancreatic bed.

Damage control for the distal pancreas is hemostasis and drainage

---

The kidneys

Access and vascular control

At laparotomy, the injured kidney typically presents as a lateral retroperitoneal (perinephric) hematoma (Chapter 9). Deal with a massively bleeding kidney in an unstable patient by rapid mobilization and control of the vascular pedicle, just like you deal with the injured spleen. A

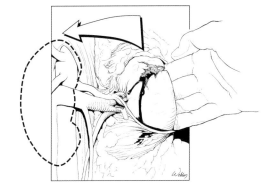

medial visceral rotation (Chapter 4) on the left or on the right gives you rapid access to the injured kidney. Incise Gerota's fascia laterally and lift the kidney out of its bed. Now you can pinch the hilum with your fingers and carefully place a vascular clamp across it to control the bleeding. The obvious similarity to the spleen is striking.

Bring a massively bleeding kidney to the midline

If you must explore a perinephric hematoma in a stable patient, you can gain vascular control of the renal vessels at their origin by using a maneuver called *midline looping*. With this maneuver, you obtain proximal control prior to entering the hematoma, but at the price of tedious dissection. The first moves are essentially those of infrarenal aortic exposure. Eviscerate the small bowel and pull it up and to the right. Take down the ligament of Treitz and open the posterior peritoneum

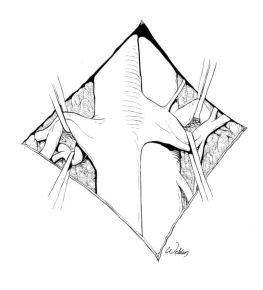

overlying the aorta. First, identify the LRV crossing in front of the aorta beneath the inferior border of the pancreas and encircle it with a vessel loop. This is the first of four loopings. Very gently retract the LRV downward (without avulsing the adrenal, left gonadal or lumbar veins that branch off it), and you will gain access to the left renal artery taking off from the aorta behind and above the LRV. Pass your second vessel loop around it.

Midline looping is trickier on the right. You must first identify and loop the short right renal vein; then, dissect in the window between it and the IVC to loop the right renal artery as it emerges from behind the IVC. All this is time-consuming and opens the door to potential pitfalls. We consider it a long run for a short slide and rarely use it. You can easily get by without it if you remember to rapidly lift the injured kidney to the midline, just as you do with the spleen.

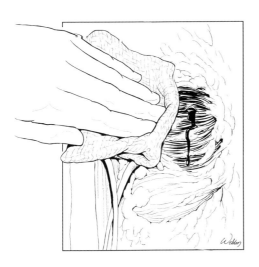

What are the damage control options for renal trauma? One obvious option is *not* to explore the kidney. If the perinephric hematoma is stable and non-expanding, leave it alone. If you see oozing but no massive hemorrhage through a hole in Gerota's fascia, pack the kidney. Remember that urine extravasation is much less ominous than leaking intestinal content (Chapter 4).

If the kidney is bleeding massively and is obviously not amenable to reconstruction, or has a hilar vascular injury in conjunction with other life-threatening injuries, a rapid nephrectomy is lifesaving. Lift the mobilized kidney up, identify the artery and vein, suture-ligate the artery and tie off the vein. Then, divide the ureter between ligatures and put the kidney in the bucket.

When considering your options, always think about the contralateral kidney. You will go the extra mile and invest additional effort in renal preservation if you know that the patient does not have another functioning kidney. If you do not have preoperative imaging to prove a functioning renal mass on the other side, what should you do? An on-table intravenous pyelogram to prove the presence of a functioning contralateral renal mass is one option. This takes time and often yields an irritating fuzzogram rather than a satisfactory image. A better option is to palpate the other kidney. If it feels normal in size and consistency and the patient is making urine despite a hilar clamp across the injured kidney, the risk of postoperative renal dysfunction is very small.

Palpate the contralateral kidney

Repair options for the injured kidney cover a wide spectrum, ranging from application of topical hemostatic agent to extracorporeal bench repair with autotransplantation. The best advice we can give you is - don't use them. Call a urologist in to repair the kidney. An experienced urologist is more likely to achieve a good result, will follow the patient, and manage any complications.

Repair of renal vascular injuries (both blunt or penetrating) is much less common and more challenging than the trauma literature leads you to believe. On the right side, penetrating hilar injuries are typically part of wounds to the *surgical soul*, one of the most devastating combinations of injuries in trauma surgery (Chapter 8). The proximity of the renal hilum to the IVC means that a penetrating injury will involve both the renal artery and the IVC or other adjacent structures like the pancreaticoduodenal complex. Injury to the short right renal vein is essentially a side-hole in the IVC, for which the prime concern is control of life-threatening hemorrhage, not renal salvage. On the left, don't hesitate to ligate the renal vein if it is injured proximal to its gonadal and adrenal branches. The Mattox maneuver (Chapter 4) gives you excellent access to the left renal artery.

When dealing with an ischemic kidney after blunt trauma in a stable patient, your decision to revascularize the kidney hinges on the time elapsed since injury, presence of functioning contralateral kidney, the patient's overall trauma burden, and available expertise. Many of these injuries are amenable to endovascular stenting. Never jeopardize the patient's life to save a kidney.

If you are fixing an injured renal artery, perfuse the kidney intermittently with iced heparinized saline and choose the simplest repair option. If the artery can be repaired end-to-end, go for it. More often, you have to interpose a graft. The graft of choice is probably a reversed saphenous vein, but the most expeditious option is a 6mm ePTFE conduit. Hook it up to the renal artery (distal anastomosis) first because this allows you better access to the posterior wall of the anastomosis. Choose a convenient location on the lateral aspect of the infrarenal aorta, control it with a side-biting clamp, and do a small aortotomy. Trim the graft and complete the proximal anastomosis to the aortotomy in an end-to-side configuration.

> **Don't kill the patient while trying to save a kidney**

THE KEY POINTS

▶   The spleen, kidney, and tail of the pancreas are take-outable.

▶   Mobilize the spleen to unlock the left upper quadrant.

▶   Do what it takes to bring the spleen to the midline.

▶   For splenic repair, consider trauma burden, age, injury, and experience.

▶   Stay close to the spleen.

▶   Don't persist if splenorrhaphy doesn't work.

▶   Look at the pancreas from the front - but mobilize it from the left.

▶   You don't need photographs to deal with a pancreatic injury.

▶   Damage control for the distal pancreas is hemostasis and drainage.

▶   Bring a massively bleeding kidney to the midline.

▶   Palpate the contralateral kidney.

▶   Don't kill the patient while trying to save a kidney.

Chapter 8

The Wounded Surgical Soul

Medical illustrators are optimists.

~ Matthew J. Wall, Jr., MD

It's difficult to imagine a more unwelcome sight during laparotomy for penetrating trauma than a large hematoma or vigorous bleeding from the right upper quadrant beneath the liver. If this is what you see, you have just been dealt one of the worst possible hands in the trauma game. We call these injuries the *wounded surgical soul*. According to tradition in our hospital, the seat of the soul of the injured patient is a spherical area, not much larger than a silver dollar, centered on the head of the pancreas. They are called soul wounds because they are more lethal than any other type of abdominal trauma.

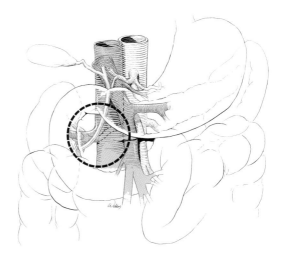

A gunshot to the surgical soul commands the greatest respect from trauma surgeons because it frequently leads to intraoperative exsanguination. You may initially encounter a contained or slowly expanding hematoma that doesn't look particularly ominous. But once you open it and unroof the underlying major vascular injuries, the demons are unleashed and the patient exsanguinates in your hands. Another unwelcome surprise is when a novice pokes an exploring finger into a soul wound, only to face torrential hemorrhage when the probing finger is withdrawn. Why are these injuries so problematic?

First, consider the vascular anatomy of the area. The portal vein, the superior mesenteric vessels, the pancreaticoduodenal arcade, the IVC and the right renal pedicle all converge at the surgical soul. Since some of these vessels directly overlay each other, a penetrating injury typically involves more than one major vessel. Now consider accessibility. The neck of the pancreas overlies the portal vein confluence and the proximal superior mesenteric vessels. The pancreatic head and duodenal loop (referred to in this chapter as the pancreaticoduodenal complex) cover the IVC and right renal pedicle. So, none of the vessels is easily accessible. The situation has worst-case scenario written all over it. A disciplined and priority-oriented approach is your only hope.

Immediate concerns

Your first priority with soul wounds is to control hemorrhage. Always assume that bleeding is from more than one major vascular injury until proven otherwise. The major bleeding sources around the surgical soul are arranged in three layers: deep, middle, and superficial.

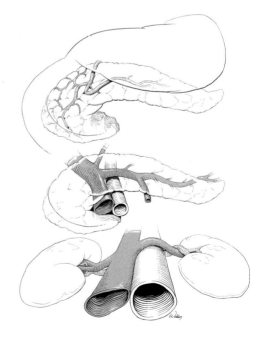

1. The *deep layer* includes the IVC and the right renal pedicle. You will see a rapidly expanding right-sided retroperitoneal hematoma or active bleeding from the area of the right renal hilum. Pack or manually compress it. Don't unroof it.

2. The *middle layer* includes the retropancreatic vessels: the superior mesenteric artery (SMA) and vein (SMV), and the portal vein. The secret of temporary bleeding control is rapid mobilization with a Kocher

maneuver (Chapter 4). If bleeding is from the root of the mesentery below (caudal to) the pancreas, control it by insinuating your left hand behind the root of the mesentery and pinching it between thumb and forefinger. If the source of bleeding is behind the pancreas, manually compress the entire pancreaticoduodenal complex. Temporarily control bleeding from the hepatoduodenal ligament by pinching the portal triad (Chapter 6).

3. The *superficial layer* consists of the injured pancreaticoduodenal complex itself. Injury to the head of the pancreas can be the source of brisk bright-red bleeding from the pancreaticoduodenal vessels. Here again, the quickest way to gain temporary control is a Kocher maneuver, which enables you to compress the entire pancreaticoduodenal complex in your hands or encircle it with a Penrose drain to get temporary hemostasis.

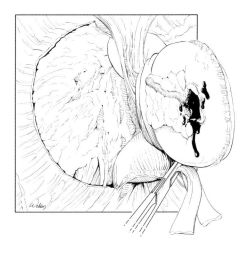

Some soul wounds bleed freely into the peritoneal cavity, while others present as a contained hematoma. Control of free bleeding comes first. Never ever "poke a skunk" by entering a contained hematoma until all free bleeding has been controlled and you have organized your attack.

Supraceliac aortic clamping is a useful adjunct in a crashing patient. Double clamping of both the supraceliac and infrarenal aorta (to control backflow) helps reduce bleeding from injuries to the superior mesenteric vessels and the portal vein but will not dry up the operative field.

All this seems nice and neat when sitting at home reading (or writing) about it. But the professional term for what you meet in real life is *multifocal exsanguination*, rapid bleeding from multiple sources, none of them easy to control. A less professional term is bloody mess, and you have no time to consult www.bloodymess.org for advice. You must staunch the bleeding NOW using a combination of packing, the Kocher maneuver, manual pressure, and careful clamping.

Once you have gained temporary control of hemorrhage, stop the operation and organize your attack on the injury. Don't just dive in without appropriate instruments, plenty of blood units in the OR, an auto-transfusion device, a rapid infuser, optimal exposure, and competent help. Bleeding from a soul wound takes BIG TROUBLE (Chapter 2) to a new level - TREMENDOUS TROUBLE.

Soul wounds bleed from more than one vascular injury

Improving exposure

The key to anything you may need to do around the surgical soul is the widest possible Kocher maneuver (Chapter 4). For bleeding from the deep layer (IVC and right kidney), extend the Kocher maneuver into a full right-sided medial visceral rotation by mobilizing the right colon and

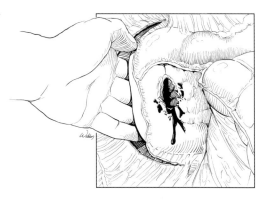

retract the liver cephalad to create a work space around the pararenal IVC. If the right renal hilum is involved, mobilizing the right kidney out of Gerota's fascia and rotating it medially helps you gain control of the hilum.

Use the Cattell-Braasch maneuver (Chapter 4) to obtain the widest possible exposure of the surgical soul. This maneuver uncovers the third and fourth parts of the duodenum, allows you to reach the proximal SMA and SMV as they emerge beneath the neck of the pancreas, and even gives you some access to the retropancreatic portal vein.

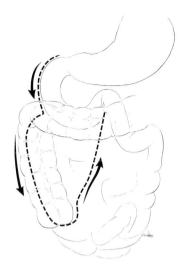

> **Use the Cattell-Braasch maneuver to expose the surgical soul**

The supraduodenal portal vein

Injury to the supraduodenal portal vein is usually associated with a high-grade liver injury and presents as a hematoma in the hepatoduodenal ligament. The *Double Pringle* maneuver is the textbook-recommended

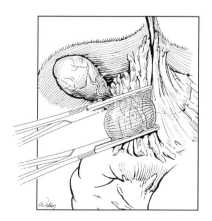

technique for definitive control of injury to the portal triad, including the supraduodenal portion of the portal vein. Begin with a Kocher maneuver; then, coming from the right hand side, place one vascular clamp immediately above the upper border of the duodenum. Place a second vascular clamp across the portal triad, as high as possible toward the liver hilum. This allows you to open the serosa of the hepato-duodenal ligament and carefully dissect to define the injury. Unfortunately, the hepatoduodenal ligament is often too short to accommodate two clamps. A good alternative is pinching the injured area with your left hand while dissecting above and below the injury with your right.

Always assess all three elements of the portal triad because their close proximity makes it very likely that more than one structure has been hit. A stab typically causes a clean laceration of the portal vein and is amenable to lateral repair. In contrast, gunshot injuries cause massive destruction (usually in conjunction with a liver injury), requiring a complex repair such as a patch or interposition graft, which is rarely feasible in the harsh reality of multifocal exsanguination.

The damage control solution for a complex supraduodenal portal vein injury is ligation. It is a realistic option and compatible with survival if the hepatic artery is intact. When both portal vein and hepatic artery are injured, you have to reconstruct one of them.

> **Ligation is the bail out solution for portal vein injury**

The retropancreatic vessels

Injuries to the retropancreatic vessels (the confluence of the superior mesenteric and splenic veins, as well as the retropancreatic part of the SMA) are particularly lethal because you can't get to them. Pancreatic transection across the neck exposes these injuries. One of us finds this technique useful and lifesaving, while the other avoids dividing the neck of the pancreas unless the injury has done it for him.

To transect the pancreas, compress the bleeding pancreaticoduodenal complex with your left hand to temporarily control the bleeding. Do a complete Cattell-Braasch maneuver to optimize access to the complex from all sides. Rapidly create a retropancreatic tunnel by opening the hepatoduodenal ligament and bluntly dissecting immediately to the left, anterior to the common bile duct, and behind the pancreatic neck. Transect the neck of the pancreas using the cautery over your finger, but avoid pushing instruments (clamps or staplers) into the tunnel because they may aggravate a retropancreatic portal vein injury. Cutting the pancreas brings you face-to-face with the injured large vein underneath, giving you an opportunity to fix it. Control bleeding from the edges of the transected pancreas (or from adjacent bleeders) only after you have controlled the injured portal vein.

If possible, do a lateral repair of the retropancreatic veins. However, if you end up with a ligated (or oversewn) portal vein and a live patient, take a deep breath and congratulate yourself.

> **Transect the pancreas to gain access to the portal vein confluence**

The root of the mesentery

While pinching the bleeding root of the mesentery between thumb and forefinger, lift the transverse colon cephalad and pull the small bowel caudally and to the left. This stretches the mesentery of the small bowel. Make a transverse incision in the serosa of the root of the mesentery and carefully dissect in the mesenteric hematoma to find the SMA and SMV, define the injury, and clamp it selectively.

If the injury is immediately below the pancreatic border, optimize your exposure by mobilizing the ligament of Treitz or by doing a full Cattell-Braasch maneuver. The SMA is exposed, allowing you to place your clamps selectively. Never clamp blindly at the root of the mesentery - it is a recipe for disaster.

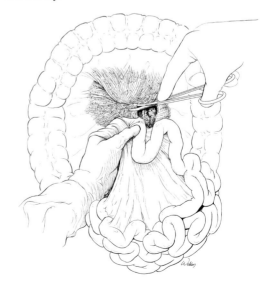

Reconstruction of the SMA is discussed in the next chapter. Repair the injured SMV if you can; if not, ligate it. Following ligation of either the portal vein or the SMV, the inevitable consequence is massive fluid sequestration and midgut edema, which translate into extremely high postoperative fluid requirements and an inability to close the abdomen. In fact, as we wrote this chapter, a patient of ours with a soul wound underwent SMV ligation. His vacuum pack drained 16 (!) liters of serous fluid from the peritoneal cavity on the first postoperative day. Don't forget that venous gangrene of the bowel is a distinct threat, so always do a second look laparotomy to ascertain bowel viability.

Blind clamping at the root of the mesentery is a recipe for disaster

---

The pancreaticoduodenal complex

Some of the most fascinating reading in the trauma literature describes pancreaticoduodenal repair techniques, spanning a wide range of very imaginative resections and reconstructions. We are particularly fond of the optimistic illustration of both ends of a transected pancreas plugged into a Roux-en-Y loop of bowel, creating two adjacent pancreaticojejunostomies and proving that the printed page tolerates anything. Unfortunately, patients don't.

Keep things as simple as possible, avoid acrobatics, and stick to a limited menu of straightforward options. You will not find a detailed exposition of all possible pancreaticoduodenal reconstructive techniques in this chapter. Instead, we give you a very limited menu of simple and safe techniques that work for us. Three cardinal principles should guide your approach to proximal pancreatic and duodenal injuries:

1. Drain every suture line in the duodenum and every significant pancreatic injury.
2. Provide a route for enteral feeding distal to the duodenum. For minor injuries, a nasojejunal tube is an option. In major trauma, a feeding jejunostomy provides a critical "nutritional safety valve" for your patient.
3. Most importantly, choose your repair technique based not on how well it works, but on how well it *fails* (Chapter 1).

Choose your repair based on how well it fails

Duodenal injuries

Can you close the injured duodenum without tension? In most cases, definitive repair of a duodenal laceration is a simple lateral suture. Just as in small bowel injuries, orient your suture line transversely, even if the laceration is longitudinal, to avoid narrowing the lumen. If the laceration is too long to achieve a transverse repair without tension, do a longitudinal repair. The suture technique is a matter of personal preference. We usually do a single layer continuous repair in an inverting fashion.

The problematic wounds are inside the duodenal loop on the pancreatic aspect of the wall, where precise visualization of the laceration is difficult. As in other situations where the injured posterior wall of a structure is inaccessible, consider opening the duodenum and repairing the injury from the inside.

Protect any duodenal repair that is more than a straightforward short suture line with a pyloric exclusion. This is good advice for suture lines that are long, multiple, delayed, or appear tenuous. Some surgeons decompress duodenal repairs either by a lateral duodenostomy or by inserting a retrograde tube from the proximal jejunum as part of a 3-tube system that also includes a gastrostomy and a feeding jejunostomy. We don't routinely do a tube duodenostomy, but we drain all duodenal repairs externally with a closed suction drain.

What if the duodenum is nearly transected? In the 1st, 3rd and 4th parts, you may be able to carefully debride the duodenal wall to healthy tissue and then do an end-to-end anastomosis. With the very limited mobility that you have, it is easiest to begin sewing on the pancreatic side, working your way around the duodenal circumference from within the lumen. However, in the duodenal loop, the adherence of the pancreas and the proximity of the ampulla usually preclude a duodenoduodenostomy.

The most versatile reconstructive option for large duodenal defects is bringing up a Roux-en-Y loop of jejunum to repair the defect or to re-establish GI continuity. Keep in mind, however, a Roux-en-Y reconstruction is time-consuming and relevant only in a stable patient with no other active injuries. Since severe duodenal trauma is almost always associated with other injuries, we use the Roux-en-Y technique mostly for delayed reconstructions, very rarely during the initial operation.

There are no good damage control options for a bad injury to the 2nd part of the duodenum. If you need to bail out quickly, approximate the edges of a large defect around an external drain to convert the open duodenum into a controlled fistula. This should be an absolutely last resort, since repairing the duodenal injury is always a much better option.

Repair inaccessible duodenal injuries from the inside

Pancreatic injuries

What are the damage control options for injuries to the head of the pancreas? For a non-bleeding injury, the quick and simple solution is external drainage, converting even a major duct disruption into a controlled pancreatic fistula that has a surprisingly benign natural course.

Bleeding from a proximal pancreatic injury requires careful assessment. Once the pancreaticoduodenal complex has been mobilized by a Kocher maneuver, control bleeding by local pressure, hemostatic sutures, or packing. Unless the entire pancreaticoduodenal complex is shattered, massive hemorrhage from a proximal pancreatic injury is always from an underlying major vascular injury.

Don't fiddle with the pancreas! The classic teaching is to establish the presence of a major pancreatic duct injury. Reality is somewhat different. Intraoperative examination of the injury will seldom provide an answer, and you are already familiar with our lack of enthusiasm for on-table pancreatography (Chapter 7). The truth is that it probably doesn't matter whether the duct is injured or not because external drainage works well in either case.

Don't fiddle with the pancreas - drain it!

Those who like playing with dynamite adhere to the traditional concept of preserving pancreatic tissue. What it amounts to is performing a pancreaticojejunostomy on a normal pancreatic stump, a high-risk anastomosis even under the best elective circumstances. Consider, for example, the options for fracture of the neck of the pancreas, where the gland is transected by an anteroposterior impact against the spine. The safest definitive option for this injury is closure of the proximal stump, followed by resecting the distal pancreas or oversewing the open distal stump. Anatomical reconstruction would mean debridement of the stump and dunking a normal soft pancreatic remnant into a Roux-en-Y loop of bowel, in close proximity to an oversewn pancreatic head and a bowel suture line. If this sounds unsafe to you, we agree. While enthusiastically described in textbooks and often discussed, current reports of what surgeons actually do (as opposed to what they talk about) indicate this approach is very rarely used. Apparently, enough surgeons have learned the painful lesson that fiddling with the traumatized pancreas does not pay. We prefer to close the pancreatic stump and drain it.

> **Avoid pancreaticojejunostomy for trauma**

Combined injuries

Bleeding patients with combined injuries to the pancreas and duodenum do not die from a duodenal leak - they exsanguinate. So stop the bleeding and bail out. If you can rapidly close the duodenum, do it. Otherwise, use a combination of external drainage and ligation to control duodenal, biliary, and pancreatic content. Return for a later reconstruction if the patient makes it.

Pyloric exclusion is an effective technique for temporarily diverting the gastric content away from the injured pancreaticoduodenal complex. Being Baylor surgeons, we have a bias toward this elegant procedure we learned from George L. Jordan, Jr., who conceived it. We advise using it to protect duodenal suture lines in combined pancreaticoduodenal injuries where the duodenum can be closed and the ampulla is intact.

After repairing the duodenal injury, identify the pylorus and make a longitudinal gastrotomy on the anterior surface of the antrum, close to the pylorus. Through the gastrotomy, palpate the pyloric ring with your finger, grasp it with a Babcock clamp, and pull it toward you. Oversew the pyloric ring with a heavy (size 0) suture on a large needle, taking big bites. We use a monofilament

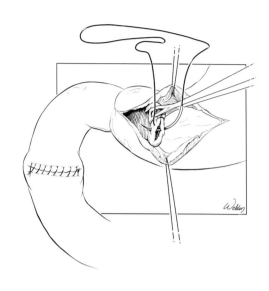

suture, but regardless of the suture material, the pylorus opens in 2-4 weeks. In fact, you can staple across the pylorus using a linear stapler with the same result.

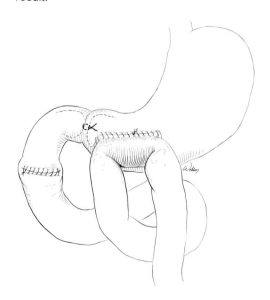

Once the pylorus is closed, bring up a loop of proximal jejunum and do a gastrojejunostomy. The last step in the procedure is providing a route for enteral feeding into the jejunum. The operation is not ulcerogenic, and vagotomy is not part of it.

The Achilles heel of pyloric exclusion is the gastroenterostomy since it carries a significant risk of non-function. To avoid this problem, some surgeons prefer to do pyloric exclusion without gastroenterostomy, relying on distal enteral feeding until the pylorus opens.

Use pyloric exclusion to protect complicated duodenal suture lines

---

The "Ultimate Big Whack"

A trauma Whipple is the ultimate big whack of abdominal trauma. Use it as a last resort when the pancreaticoduodenal complex is destroyed or when the ampulla cannot be reconstructed and no simpler solution will work. It is often said that you should consider a trauma Whipple when the injury has already done most of the dissection for you. Herein lies the big paradox of this operation: the exsanguinating patient with a shattered pancreaticoduodenal complex is too sick to survive it. A stable patient who will survive it often does not need it. So choose a lesser alternative, however imperfect, whenever you can.

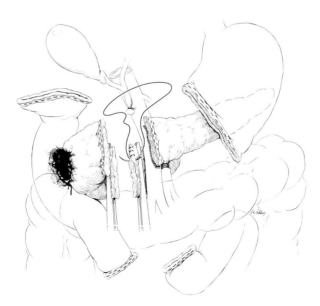

The three important differences between a Whipple for trauma and a Whipple for cancer are: dissecting the uncinate process, removing the gallbladder, and staged reconstruction.

♦ During the resection stage for trauma, don't dissect the uncinate process off the SMV and the SMA. Leave most of it adherent to the SMV by dividing it piecemeal and oversewing it with a running stitch for hemostasis as you proceed. This greatly simplifies one of the tricky steps of the dissection.

♦ Think twice before removing the gallbladder in a trauma patient. A fine and delicate common bile duct may force you to use the gallbladder for the biliary-enteric reconstruction.

♦ The most important difference is that a trauma Whipple is a staged procedure. During the initial damage control operation, achieve hemostasis and do the resection, not the reconstruction. Leave the stomach, jejunum, and pancreatic stump stapled off. Leave the common bile duct ligated or drained. At reoperation, perform the anastamoses. Except under the most favorable circumstances, we leave the distal pancreatic stump stapled or oversewn and do not join it to the bowel (or to the stomach) to avoid a high-risk anastomosis in a critically ill patient.

> **If forced to do a trauma Whipple - do it in stages**

Putting it all together

We hope you realize by now why injuries to the surgical soul deserve a special chapter. The strategic dimension of a soul wound is straightforward, since it is pretty obvious from the very beginning that you must operate in damage control mode and dart out of the belly as quickly as you possibly can. The challenge of soul wounds lies in their tactical complexity. You must simplify the tactical situation (Chapter 1). Ask yourself which elements of the problem can be rapidly eliminated. Look at the deep layer of bleeding from the IVC and right renal pedicle. Do you really intend to do a complex vascular repair of this bleeding renal pedicle in the context of multifocal exsanguination? Of course not. On the other hand, a swift nephrectomy will open the way to the IVC injury.

Are you going to hook the pancreatic stump to bowel as the patient is getting the 34th unit of blood? You must be kidding! A rapid distal pancreatectomy, however, may enable you to reach the left side of the retropancreatic portal vein.

These examples show you how to simplify tactical situations. Constantly ask yourself what the simplest solution is for a specific injury - and go for it. The only hope for a patient with a soul wound is a surgeon who thinks about ligation, resection, drainage, and shunting - not about spiral vein grafts and Roux-en-Y pancreaticojejunostomies.

> **Look for ways to simplify the tactical situation**

THE KEY POINTS

▶ Soul wounds bleed from more than one vascular injury.

▶ Use the Cattell-Braasch maneuver to expose the surgical soul.

▶ Ligation is the bail out solution for portal vein injury.

▶ Transect the pancreas to gain access to the portal vein confluence.

▶ Blind clamping at the root of the mesentery is a recipe for disaster.

▶ Choose your repair based on how well it fails.

▶ Repair inaccessible duodenal injuries from the inside.

▶ Don't fiddle with the pancreas - drain it!

▶ Avoid pancreaticojejunostomy for trauma.

▶   Use pyloric exclusion to protect complicated duodenal suture lines.

▶   If forced to do a trauma Whipple - do it in stages.

▶   Look for ways to simplify the tactical situation.

Chapter 9
Big Red & Big Blue:
Abdominal Vascular Trauma

...Upon entering the peritoneal cavity, approximately 2 to 3 liters of blood, both liquid and in clots, were encountered. These were removed. The bullet pathway was then identified as having shattered the upper medial surface of the spleen, then entered the retroperitoneal area where there was a large retroperitoneal hematoma in the area of the pancreas. Following this, bleeding seemed to be coming from the right side, and upon inspection there was seen to be an exit to the right through the inferior vena cava, thence through the superior pole of the right kidney, the lower portion of the right lobe of the liver, and into the right lateral body wall... The inferior vena cava hole was clamped with a partial occlusion clamp... The inspection of the retroperitoneal area revealed a huge hematoma in the midline. The spleen was then mobilized, as was the left colon, and the retroperitoneal approach was made to the mid-line structures. The pancreas was seen to be shattered in its mid portion, bleeding was seen to be coming from the aorta... Bleeding was controlled by finger pressure by Dr. Malcolm O. Perry. Upon identification of this injury, the superior mesenteric artery had been sheared off the aorta... This was clamped with a small, curved DeBakey clamp. The aorta was then occluded with a straight DeBakey clamp above and a Potts clamp below. At this point all major bleeding was controlled... Shortly thereafter... the pulse rate... was found to be 40 and a few seconds later found to be zero. No pulse was felt in the aorta at this time.

~ Operative Record of Lee Harvey Oswald,
Parkland Memorial Hospital 11/24/63
Cited in: *The Warren Commission Report: Report of the President's Commission on the Assassination of President John F. Kennedy*,
St Martin's Press, 1992

No author has ever captured the tremendous challenge and unforgiving nature of abdominal vascular trauma better than this dry, technical operative report describing G. Tom Shires and his team at Parkland doing battle with multiple vascular injuries in the abdomen of Lee Harvey Oswald. The report emphasizes the central features of abdominal vascular trauma: massive bleeding from inaccessible sites, multiple associated injuries, and an extremely narrow window of opportunity to save the patient. You not only see the bleeding, but you can also often hear it. Because the patient is exsanguinating, you rarely have time to summon a more experienced colleague to help you gain control. You have to fasten your seat belt and get going.

The "rules of engagement"

An abdominal vascular injury presents as free intraperitoneal hemorrhage, retroperitoneal hematoma or, most commonly, a combination of both. In either case, it is always BIG TROUBLE, and the key to success is temporary control followed by a well-organized attack. The location of the hematoma dictates the operative approach.

Operative Approach to Retroperitoneal Hematoma

Hematoma	Explore?		Proximal control	Key maneuver
	Penetrating	Blunt		
Midline supramesocolic	Yes	Yes	Supraceliac aorta	Mattox maneuver
Midline inframesocolic	Yes	Yes	Infrarenal aorta or IVC	Infrarenal aortic exposure or right-sided visceral rotation
Lateral perinephric	Selective	No	Hilar clamping or midline looping	Mobilize kidney
Pelvic	Yes	No	Distal aorta/ IVC	"Walking the clamps"

Midline supramesocolic hematoma

All midline supramesocolic hematomas must be explored. If the patient is in shock or if you see rapid active hemorrhage from the supramesocolic area, manually compress the supraceliac aorta (Chapter 2). If the patient is hemodynamically stable, begin with the Mattox maneuver. The medial visceral rotation allows you to gain proximal control of the lower thoracic aorta by cutting the left crus of the diaphragm (Chapter 4). Always obtain distal control above the aortic bifurcation because without it, considerable back bleeding will obscure the injury.

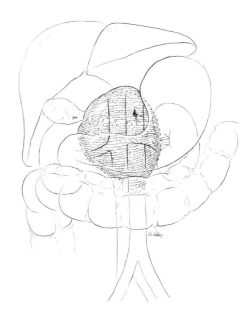

Injuries to the paravisceral aortic segment between the celiac and the renal arteries are highly lethal. They are always associated with injuries to adjacent structures. Blood loss is typically massive, control is not straightforward, and repair requires supraceliac clamping. For all these reasons, try to get away with a lateral repair if you can.

If you must sew in a synthetic interposition graft, you are obviously racing against the renal ischemic time, and the patient's chances of making it are not great. Select a knitted Dacron graft that is slightly larger than the aortic diameter because the aorta of a young patient in shock is vasoconstricted. Since you have no alternative, don't hesitate to put in a graft even in the presence of intestinal spillage. There are no effective damage control options for these injuries. The patient's only hope is a rapid definitive repair of the aorta and bail out solutions for associated injuries.

Try to get away with lateral repair in suprarenal aortic injuries

Pentrating trauma to the proximal renal artery is essentially a side-hole in the aorta. Initial control and exposure are the same as previously described above. The realistic options for definitive repair or damage control of the renal vessels were described in Chapter 7.

Injury to the celiac axis or its branches is uncommon - but deadly. Typically, you see a gastric injury with either an expanding hematoma behind the stomach or brisk arterial bleeding from behind and above the lesser curve. This is one of the toughest and least advertised situations in abdominal trauma.

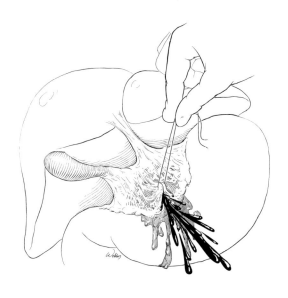

While you can gain proximal control of the celiac axis by medial visceral rotation, this will not help you see or control bleeding from its branches. Furthermore, the operative circumstances may force you to attack the bleeder from the front. There are no standard prepackaged solutions for this difficult situation. A technique that has worked for us is inserting a gross hemostatic stitch with a heavy suture on a big needle (such as size 0 polypropylene) into the lesser omentum above the lesser curve of the stomach and suturing until the bleeding stops.

A useful alternative is transecting the stomach by firing a linear cutting stapler across the body, giving you immediate access to the vascular injury behind it. If the patient survives, complete the hemigastrectomy at reoperation. Dissecting out the origin of the celiac axis, encased in a thick layer of periaortic tissue, is not a realistic option in a bleeding patient.

Injury to the proximal SMA is another unforgiving situation that presents as a midline supramesocolic hematoma. An injury to the SMA above the pancreas is essentially an anterior hole in the suprarenal aorta. Control it from the left side by performing a Mattox maneuver and clamping the aorta above and below the take-off of the vessel. You can then get to the injured SMA, either from the side or front, by making a hole in the lesser omentum and retracting the upper border of the pancreas caudally. These injuries are typically associated with damage to the pancreas and adjacent bowel. Often your best option with a proximal SMA injury is ligation, followed by retrograde reconstruction.

Control of bleeding from the retropancreatic SMA is achieved by dividing the pancreas (Chapter 8). An injury to the SMA below the pancreas will manifest as a large hematoma at the root of the mesentery.

The damage control option for SMA injuries is inserting a temporary shunt. While we have not done it, others have reported it worked for them. Ligating the proximal SMA in a severely hypotensive and vasoconstricted patient is not a good option because it leads to bowel ischemia. So how should you reconstruct the SMA?

The principles are to use the most expedient method and stay away from the injured pancreas, because a leaking pancreas and an arterial suture line don't sit well together. To do a retrograde reconstruction from the infra-mesocolic aorta, you need access to the side or to the posterior aspect of the vessel. You can approach the SMA immediately below the pancreas and from the left by dividing the ligament of Treitz and mobilizing the fourth portion of the duodenum.

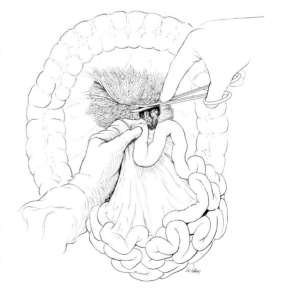

Alternatively, do a full Cattell-Braasch maneuver and reflect the small bowel upward to obtain good access to the posterior aspect of the SMA. If you are not sure how to do it, you can dissect out a more distal (and therefore smaller) segment of the SMA at the base of the mesentery.

Reconstruct the injured SMA using a 6mm ringed ePTFE graft from the distal aorta or the right common iliac artery. Using the latter has advantages: it does not require aortic clamping, is easy to cover with omentum, and is technically straightforward.

> **Reconstruct the SMA away from the injured pancreas**

Midline inframesocolic hematoma

Eviscerate the small bowel to the right, pull the transverse colon upward, and take a good look at the retroperitoneal hematoma waiting in the shadows. If the bulk of the hematoma is to the left of the small bowel mesentery, you probably are dealing with an infrarenal aortic injury that can be approached through the midline. If, however, the hematoma is more to the right, pushing on the ascending colon from behind, you probably are dealing with an IVC injury and should do a right-sided medial visceral rotation.

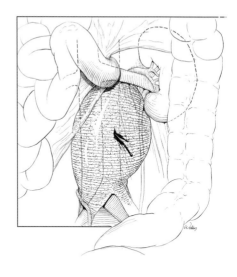

Approach an inframesocolic aortic injury as you would a ruptured aortic aneurysm. If you have time, place a self-retaining retractor and organize the operative field to keep the bowel eviscerated and out of your way. The

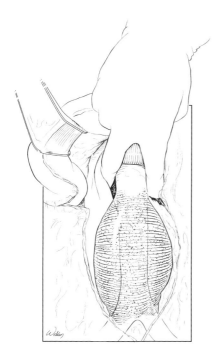

classic pitfall in proximal control of the infrarenal aorta is iatrogenic injury to the LRV or IVC. To avoid it, look at the shape and precise location of the hematoma. Is it distal, away from the root of the transverse mesocolon? If so, the risk of inadvertent injury to the LRV is small. Mobilize the ligament of Treitz, reflect the fourth portion of the duodenum laterally, and enter the safe periaortic plane. Bluntly create a space for a clamp on both sides of the aorta using your fingers. However, if the hematoma extends higher up obscuring the ligament of Treitz, it will be much safer to gain supraceliac control through the lesser omentum above the stomach, either by manually compressing the aorta against the spine or by clamping through the right crus of the diaphragm (Chapter 2).

With proximal control in place, enter the hematoma and, using blunt dissection, carefully orient yourself to avoid the LRV. Dissect distally in the periaortic plane to define the injury. Reposition your clamps below the renal arteries to control troublesome back bleeding from the distal aorta or from the lumbar arteries and begin the repair.

Beware of iatrogenic vein injury in an inframesocolic hematoma

---

Unfortunately, we cannot offer you good damage control options for the infrarenal aorta either. We have tried inserting a chest tube as a temporary shunt in extreme situations but did not have a survivor. However, in 1945, C.E. Holzer of Cincinnati bridged a large abdominal aortic defect from a gunshot wound with a vitallium tube secured with umbilical tape. The patient survived and went home with the tube in place. Another desperate measure for extreme situations is oversewing the injured infrarenal aorta and bilateral fasciotomies, followed by extra-anatomical revascularization if the patient survives the physiological insult.

What are the definitive repair options? Unless the laceration is small and amenable to simple lateral repair, your best bet is to grab the bull by the horns and insert a short 14-18mm synthetic interposition graft. Since the aorta of healthy young patients is small and tears easily, attempts to sew in a patch or do an end-to-end anastomosis often lead to an unsatisfactory result. We advise you save yourself grief and go directly for graft interposition using knitted Dacron.

Always cover your inframesocolic vascular suture lines with omentum. Our preferred technique is to take down the greater omentum from the tranverse colon along the bloodless line, create an opening in the transverse mesocolon to the left of the middle colic artery, and swing the mobilized omentum through this hole into the inframesocolic compartment to cover the aortic reconstruction.

If you see a bleeding hole in the psoas muscle, BEWARE! This deceptively simple injury is one of those traps not mentioned in the books. Whatever you do, don't dig into the muscle in search of the source. Bleeding in these cases often originates from the ascending lumbar vein or a lumbar artery. Think of it not as a small bleeder inside a muscle, but as an inaccessible side-hole in the aorta or the IVC. Instead of a direct attack, choose another hemostatic technique: stuff the hole with a local hemostatic agent, put a balloon catheter into it, or pack it with gauze. Whatever you do - don't try to identify the bleeder. Your small bleeder will rapidly bloom into a full-scale catastrophe.

Don't chase a bleeder into the psoas muscle

The Inferior Vena Cava

A large dark hematoma behind the right colon is a sign of IVC injury. This is a unique situation in trauma surgery where you may deliberately flip a controlled situation into uncontrolled calamity. The tamponade effect of the retroperitoneum may have stopped the bleeding, and you are going to unroof the injury and release the tamponade, with a real risk of making things much worse. You better be absolutely sure you know what you're doing.

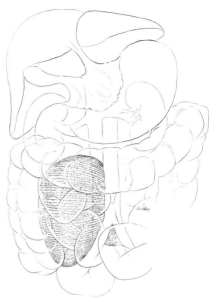

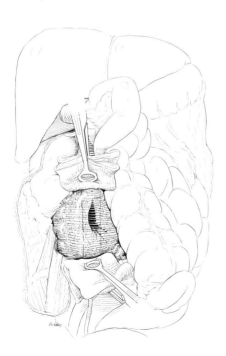

Prepare for BIG TROUBLE (Chapter 2), and then unroof the hematoma by right-sided medial visceral rotation. Once you are greeted with a violent gush of dark blood, gain temporary control by digitally compressing the IVC against the spine above and below the injury. Rapidly delegate the job to your assistant to free your hands for the repair. Digital pressure is effective, but the assistant's hands limit your work space. We prefer to use tightly rolled laparotomy pads held on ringed clamps. Watch the patient's blood pressure on the monitor, and talk to the anesthesiologist. If the patient crashes while the IVC is being controlled, compress the aorta as a hemodynamic adjunct.

The key maneuver in repairing large veins is to *define the edges* of the laceration. It is impossible to see the injury properly while the IVC is actively bleeding. You are looking for the edge of the laceration - if not all of it, at least part of it. Look for the silvery intima and gently grasp the edge of the laceration with a long hemostat or a Babcock clamp and lift it up to visualize the adjacent segment. Apply another clamp and hold it up too. As you systematically work your way around, you will

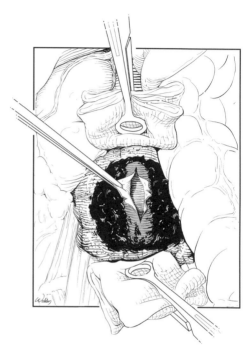

be able to define the entire circumference of the laceration and then control it with one or two vascular clamps. A side-biting Satinsky clamp is particularly useful.

Another trick is to insert a polypropylene suture at either end of the laceration and tie it while your finger occludes the hole. Gently pulling these end sutures caudad and cephalad, respectively, pulls the edges of the vein injury taut, like a rubber band or the string of a fiddle. Moving your occluding finger slowly allows you to place one suture at a time in a relatively bloodless field. Before you know it, the repair is complete.

If the IVC injury is posterior, inaccessible, or there are several lacerations, defining the edges is much more difficult. When you can see the bleeding hole but cannot define the edge or cannot apply a side-biting clamp, inserting a large Foley catheter (with a 30ml balloon) into the lumen and inflating it can help.

A hematoma behind or above the duodenal loop should warn you of a caval injury around or above the renal veins. Insert a long Deaver retractor over the inferior surface of the liver and tow in to compress the inaccossible suprarenal IVC, while simultaneously retracting the liver to provide a limited work space. Expose the right lateral and posterior aspects of the pararenal IVC by mobilizing the right kidney medially. Similarly, you can divide the proximal LRV with impunity to improve access to the left side of the IVC. Even with these maneuvers, control of the IVC at or above the renal veins is a real technical challenge.

In IVC trauma, get hold of the wound edges

What are your repair options? If the laceration is straightforward and easily accessible, do a lateral repair. If the injury requires a complex repair, the patient is stable, and you have the necessary experience, you may be tempted to engage in gymnastics. Unfortunately, this favorable combination of a complex caval injury in a stable patient with no other injuries is an extremely rare bird, almost never seen in nature. A classic example of gymnastics, an illustration you often see in books and atlases, is repair of the posterior wall of the IVC from the inside, through a longitudinal anterior venotomy. Many other neat complex reconstructive techniques have been described for high-grade caval injuries, including panel grafts, synthetic grafts, patches, and more. All belong to a branch of the trauma literature known as science fiction. They may have worked for someone somewhere, but they are not going to work for you. Our strong advice - and we cannot overemphasize this enough - is to avoid the fancy stuff. If you cannot do a simple lateral repair on the infrarenal IVC, ligate it!

Do your best to repair the actively bleeding suprarenal cava, but if the patient is *in extremis*, consider a bail out solution. Packing may work - it has certainly worked for us. Ligation is another option, accepting that the kidneys may take a hit, which is still far better than on-table exsanguination.

More importantly, if you see a non-expanding suprarenal hematoma below the liver, do not touch it. Leave it alone or pack it. Don't poke a skunk.

Ligate the IVC if lateral repair doesn't work

Pelvic hematoma

Unless you specifically suspect an iliac vascular injury, do not open a pelvic hematoma in a blunt trauma patient with a pelvic fracture. You will only make matters worse. If you find yourself facing a ruptured pelvic hematoma in such a patient, your best move is to quickly pack the pelvis, which should control venous bleeders. Follow this with a rapid temporary abdominal closure and proceed to angiography for selective embolization of arterial bleeders, typically small branches of the internal iliac arteries.

In a patient with penetrating trauma, a pelvic hematoma means injury to an iliac vessel unless proven otherwise. You must unroof the injury and fix it. If the injury is on the right, mobilize the cecum; if on the left, mobilize the sigmoid. When you can't be sure and suspect a bilateral injury, doing a full Cattell-Braasch maneuver gives you wide exposure of the iliac vessels and keeps all your options open. Now you must gain control of the pelvic vessels. Proximal control is obviously not enough. You may have forgotten the internal iliac

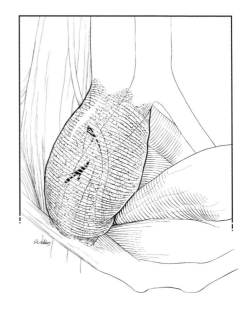

vessels, but they have not forgotten you, and they are difficult to reach. So what should you do?

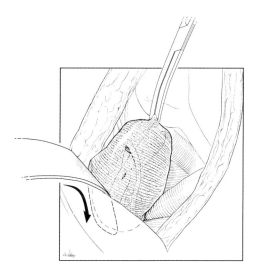

The technical principle is "walking the clamps." Begin with global control in virgin territory outside the hematoma by clamping the proximal common iliac artery together with the underlying vein. The easiest way to achieve distal control is to have your assistant tow in with a large Deaver retractor over the lower part of the open laparotomy wound, globally compressing the external iliac vessels with the retractor against the pubic bone. Now, open the posterior abdominal or pelvic peritoneum and bluntly dissect with your finger to get to the lacerated vessel. As you progress inside the hematoma, advance the clamps closer and closer to the injury, applying them to both iliac artery and vein. Initially, your control is global and remote. As you gradually converge on the source of bleeding proximally and distally, your clamping becomes more selective. Finally, isolate and control the internal iliac artery or vein using an angled vascular clamp, a Satinsky side-biting clamp, an intraluminal Fogarty balloon, or any other method that works for you.

Walking the clamps is a general technical principle that applies in any situation where an injured artery bifurcates and the deep branch is either not directly visible or inaccessible. Control of the bleeding femoral artery in the groin, carotid injuries in the neck, and penetrating trauma to the thoracic outlet are obvious examples where walking the clamps can save the day - and your patient's life.

With trauma to the aortic or caval bifurcation or when you cannot be sure which side is bleeding, you may have to do a total pelvic vascular isolation. Begin with the Cattell-Braasch maneuver to obtain the widest possible exposure of the pelvic vasculature, then proceed with clamping (or compressing) the distal aorta, and insert two Deaver retractors to compress both distal external iliac arteries and veins. Now, enter the hematoma and start walking the clamps to converge on the injuries - first on one side and then on the other. Keep in mind that the ureter passes over the bifurcation of the common iliac artery, and your patient will do so much better without a transected ureter.

Walk the clamps to gradually converge on an iliac injury

Trauma to the confluence of the common iliac veins is particularly difficult to control because it is inaccessible, lying behind the right common iliac artery. If you cannot get to it to insert a hemostatic suture, your best move is to transect the overlying right common iliac artery between clamps, giving you access to the injured confluence. If the patient survives, repair the transected artery or insert a temporary shunt.

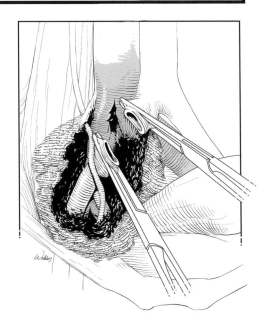

What are your repair options for the iliac vessels? By the time you have gained vascular control, the patient has typically suffered massive blood loss and has associated injuries to other abdominal organs, usually the colon, bladder or small bowel. Talk to the anesthesiologist and assess the magnitude of the physiological insult. More often than not, the situation will have damage control written all over it. If the artery requires only a simple lateral repair - just do it. If the injury is more extensive, a temporary shunt is a classic and effective bail out option.

Another alternative is to oversew the injured iliac artery, perform a fasciotomy, and watch the leg in the Surgical Intensive Care Unit (SICU). If the patient survives and the leg is grossly ischemic, do a femoro-femoral bypass to restore perfusion. If the patient is too unstable even for a trip to the OR, this straightforward bypass can be done at the bedside in SICU. The logistics can be a little demanding and the conditions awkward, but the operation is feasible and we have done it. Another useful damage control technique is to insert a Foley balloon catheter into a bleeding bullet tract deep in the pelvis to control hemorrhage from the internal iliac territory that is not accessible to direct control.

As for definitive reconstruction of an injured iliac artery, our advice is not to waste valuable time trying to mobilize a transected artery for an end-to-end repair because it rarely works. Instead, just interpose a synthetic graft.

Spillage of intestinal content is very common in iliac vascular trauma and poses a dilemma because intestinal content and synthetic grafts are not a good combination. This is, in fact, such a popular question on Board exams that you are likely to encounter it there before you face the situation in the OR. What should you do? For the Board examiners, the safest answer is also your safest option: ligate the artery and do a femoro-femoral bypass after the abdomen is closed. However, in real life we assess the degree of contamination. For limited spillage of small bowel content, it is safe to fix the bowel, irrigate the area, insert a synthetic interposition graft and cover it with omentum. If the injured iliac artery is swimming in a pool of fecal material, it doesn't take a Google search to figure out that ligation with extra-anatomic bypass is the only realistic option.

Do not dilly-dally with iliac vein injuries. They are extremely unforgiving and lethal. If you have controlled the bleeding and your patient is still alive, you have already used up a pretty large chunk of good fortune. Don't spoil everything by attempting complex repairs. If you can fix the injury with a simple lateral repair, do it. If not, ligate the vein without a moment's hesitation. The iliac veins are not mobile, so trying to close a large defect can put the repair under tension. You find yourself replacing one small hole with two larger ones. The next bite of the needle converts this into four holes, and before you know it, the game is over - you've lost. The smartest move you can make is ligate the vein.

Shunting and ligation are the bail out options for iliac artery injury

---

THE KEY POINTS

▶   Try to get away with lateral repair in suprarenal aortic injuries.

▶   Reconstruct the SMA away from the injured pancreas.

▶   Beware of iatrogenic vein injury in an inframesocolic hematoma.

▶   Don't chase a bleeder into the psoas muscle.

▶   In IVC trauma, get hold of the wound edges.

▶   Ligate the IVC if lateral repair doesn't work.

▶   Walk the clamps to gradually converge on an iliac injury.

▶   Shunting and ligation are the bail out options for iliac artery injury.

Chapter 10
Double Jeopardy:
Thoracoabdominal Injuries

*A battle is a phenomenon that always takes
place in the junction between two maps.*

~ Anonymous British Officer, 1914

Where to go first - belly or chest?

You are in the OR preparing to operate on a 17-year-old kid in severe shock. His story is very familiar: he was walking down the street minding his own business when two dudes approached and shot him in the left chest. These same two dudes pop up regularly on the streets (especially on weekend nights), shooting people who always claim they were just minding their own business. Plain x-rays of the chest and abdomen show a bullet in the epigastrium. So, the bullet went into the left chest, across the diaphragm, and into the abdomen. The chest tube you inserted on the left is actively draining blood, while the abdomen is getting noticeably distended, and the blood pressure is plummeting. Where do you begin? Chest or belly?

The clock is ticking, and your patient is bleeding. Belly or chest?

If you are unsure where to begin, you are not alone. Some of the most exasperating battles in trauma surgery occur in the junction between the abdomen and chest. During training you are likely to hear about thoracoabdominal injuries at morbidity and mortality conferences, but when you try to look them up in trauma texts, you are in for a small surprise. There is not a single chapter on thoracoabdominal trauma in any current major trauma textbook. Why? What exactly are thoracoabdominal injuries? What makes them so special?

A tour of no-man's land

The thoracoabdominal region, also known as the intrathoracic abdomen, is a unique anatomical region. It extends from the costal margin up to the nipple line anteriorly, 6th intercostal space laterally, and the tip of the scapula posteriorly. The region includes abdominal and thoracic organs on both sides of the diaphragm.

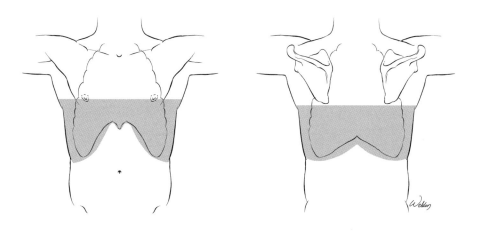

Five visceral compartments converge in the thoracoabdominal region: the right and left pleural spaces, mediastinum, upper peritoneal cavity, and upper retroperitoneum. While you are working in one compartment, lots of mischief can occur in another. A common scenario has the surgeon and entire OR team focusing on the initially selected compartment while neglecting the others. Remember also, the abdominal side of the thoracoabdominal region contains the least accessible portions of the aorta, IVC, and upper GI tract.

Five compartments converge in the thoracoabdominal region

Strategic considerations

Approximately two-thirds of patients with penetrating thoracoabdominal injuries are successfully managed by chest tube drainage followed by laparotomy (or laparoscopy). Roughly one-third will need operative intervention in both chest and abdomen, and it is in these patients that the traps await you.

Thoracoabdominal injuries are the most common form of *multicavitary* wounding, where you are dealing with bleeding in more than one visceral compartment. This is not a good situation, even for an experienced surgeon. When a wounded patient is bleeding from a single source (such as spleen or lung), you have an assortment of effective solutions to deal with the problem. But when the patient is bleeding from several sources simultaneously, you are not nearly as effective. Why? Because the physiological insult is greatly accelerated. Multiple sources of bleeding lead to quicker exsanguination; several open body cavities translate into swifter hypothermia; and you are forced to multitask between numerous areas of activity in the operative field. Lots of work to do; not enough time to do it. You must decide very quickly to switch to damage control mode. How early can you make the decision?

You may be surprised to learn that the trajectory of the bullet can help you make an early decision to bail out. A bullet trajectory across the truncal midline in a hypotensive patient is a very ominous sign because the major neurovascular bundle of the human body (aorta, vena cava, and spine) is a midline structure. Therefore, the likelihood of a major cardiovascular injury is high and so is the mortality. A trajectory across the

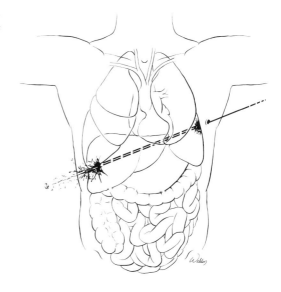

thoracoabdominal midline in a hypotensive patient should put damage control (and the possibility of a cardiac injury) foremost on your mind, even before you make the incision. We call a bullet trajectory across the truncal midline a *transaxial injury*.

In a thoracoabdominal gunshot injury, the bullet has an important story to tell, which is why surgeons with experience in penetrating trauma obtain a plain film of the chest and abdomen, if possible, before going to the OR. These radiographs, with metal markers placed adjacent to entry and exit wounds, tell you what to expect and guide you where to go.

Every bullet tells a story

Which cavity first?

When trying to decide whether to open the abdomen or chest first, you face one of the classic dilemmas of trauma surgery, and there aren't any good rules to help you. Even with a lot of trauma experience, you will begin with the *less* urgent cavity in about one-third of the cases, mainly because the chest tube output is frequently misleading. In some patients, the chest tube output actually reflects intra-abdominal hemorrhage entering the chest through a hole in the diaphragm. In others, a misplaced, kinked, or non-functioning chest tube creates a false impression that the patient is no longer bleeding. Here are some guidelines to help you decide where to go first:

◆ Be paranoid about chest tube output - it will often lead you astray. Assign a specific team member to monitor it throughout the operation.
◆ After chest tube insertion, get a chest x-ray in the ER to see if the drained side of the chest has indeed been evacuated.
◆ Have a high index of suspicion for pericardial tamponade.
◆ Use focused ultrasound (FAST). Despite obvious limitations, the FAST examination will often tell you if there is a pericardial tamponade or lots of blood in the belly.
◆ Play the odds. In a right-sided thoracoabdominal penetration, the most likely source of hemorrhage is the liver, so beginning with a laparotomy is often a good decision.

The most important advice we can offer you is to maintain tactical flexibility. Statistics show that you will often begin in one cavity while the main source of bleeding is in another. Recognize this fact and compensate for it by being vigilant and tactically flexible. Actively seek clues that something suspicious is happening on the other side of the diaphragm, like a gradually protruding hemidiaphragm progressively obscuring your operative field. Always be prepared to change your plan in mid-operation and rapidly dive into the other side of the diaphragm.

Here again, good team leadership comes into play. Talk to the anesthesiologist. Often a subtle physiological derangement or inconsistency is the only clue that hemorrhage is ongoing on the other side of the diaphragm.

Clues to Bleeding on the Other Side of the Diaphragm

Unexplained hypotension
Inappropriate response to IV fluids or blood
Gradual increase in airway pressures (sign of a hemo/pneumothorax)
Elevated central venous pressure (sign of tamponade)

Maintain tactical flexibility

Peeking into the pericardium

If you suspect a pericardial tamponade during laparotomy, the quickest way to find out is by doing a transdiaphragmatic pericardiotomy. Begin by dividing the left triangular ligament to mobilize the left lateral lobe of the liver, which usually can be folded upon itself and retracted to the right. Identify the diaphragm in the midline, anterior to the

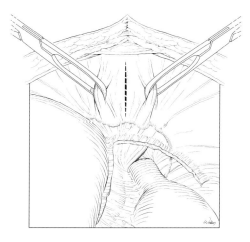

EG junction, and grasp it with two Allis clamps. Be careful not to injure the phrenic vein. Incise the diaphragm and the overlying pericardium between the Allis clamps until you see fluid escaping from the pericardial sac. If the fluid is clear, close the hole with a heavy monofilament suture. If it is bloody, proceed with either median sternotomy or left anterior thoracotomy (Chapter 11).

> **Mobilize the left lateral lobe for transdiaphragmatic pericardiotomy**

Fixing the diaphragm

Use laparoscopy to diagnose a diaphragmatic injury in asymptomatic patients with thoracoabdominal penetrations. Laparoscopy is an excellent way to look for injuries to the left diaphragm or anterior portion of the right diaphragm. If the patient doesn't have a functioning chest tube on the relevant side, insufflating the belly may cause a tension pneumothorax if there is a hole in the diaphragm. Therefore, prep and drape the chest and abdomen, and have a chest tube insertion kit ready before you begin insufflating the peritoneal cavity.

With an adequate pneumoperitoneum and the patient tilted head up, you have a nice view of the left side of the diaphragm and a partial (anterior) view of the right. If there is a diaphragmtic injury, proceed with exploratory laparotomy because you can't rely on laparoscopy to rule out a hollow organ injury. Some surgeons repair the diaphragm laparoscopically if there has been an interval of several hours from injury and the patient has remained asymptomatic.

Repair of an acute diaphragmatic laceration is usually straightforward. If there is a herniated organ in the chest, reduce it, and see if it is perforated. If you are having difficulty reducing the hernia, incise the diaphragm to enlarge the defect a little to solve your problem. When you are ready to close the laceration, grab the edges with long Allis clamps and pull them toward you. Use a clean sucker to evacuate the pleural or pericardial space above the injury. Look at the effluent in the suction

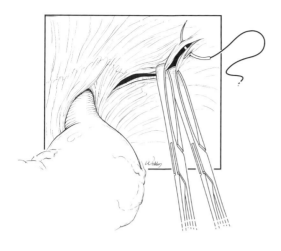

tubing. Is it clear or can you tell what the patient had for supper? If the chest is heavily contaminated, or if you are evacuating lots of blood and clot, formally open the chest to address the pleural space directly. With heavy contamination of the pleural space, trying to clean the hemithorax through the diaphragmatic defect is keyhole surgery. It is unsafe and ineffective - don't do it.

Close the diaphragmatic laceration with a non-absorbable heavy suture. We use a running suture for short lacerations and simple interrupted sutures for long ones. Some surgeons prefer horizontal mattress sutures or even a two-layer repair. An important technical principle is to leave the ends of every suture long and use them as handles to pull the diaphragmatic defect toward you. The edges of a diaphragmatic defect tend to

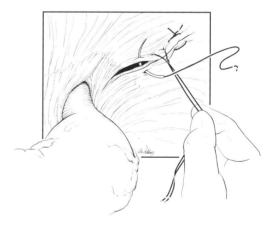

invert, so pulling on the last stitch when placing the next one will help you achieve good apposition. Take large bites to prevent bleeding from the phrenic vessels on the pleural side of the diaphragm.

What if the defect is large and you cannot approximate it with a simple suture? If the diaphragm is avulsed peripherally, as sometimes seen in severe blunt trauma, and the patient is stable, you may be able to reattach the avulsed diaphragm to a rib, usually 1-2 ribs above the level of the original avulsion. When reattachment is not an option and the defect is too large for primary repair, a non-absorbable prosthetic mesh is a quick and easy solution.

If you have to bail out or the operative field is heavily contaminated, reconstruction with synthetic non-absorbable mesh is not an option. While there is no compelling reason to close a large diaphragmatic defect when operating in damage control mode, failure to do so will force you to deal with an even larger defect at reoperation. The muscular edges of the defect rapidly retract, progressively enlarging the gap. Prevent this from happening by inserting an absorbable mesh as a temporary physical barrier between the abdomen and chest. At reoperation, if the field is clean, the absorbable mesh can be replaced by a permanent non-absorbable prosthesis.

> **When fixing the diaphragm, pull it toward you**

Opening Pandora's Box

Think twice (and possibly three times) before deciding to mobilize the liver in a patient with a thoraco-abdominal injury. You may be blowing the lid off Pandora's Box. A patient with a right-sided thoracoabdominal injury draining large amounts of dark blood from a medial hole in the diaphragm is likely to have a retrohepatic venous injury draining into the chest through the diaphragmatic defect. Going into the

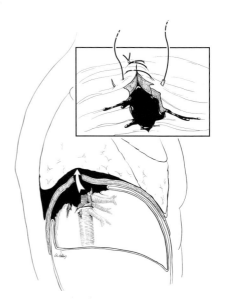

abdomen to mobilize the liver and fix the hole from below is a lethal mistake. If indeed you are dealing with a contained retrohepatic caval injury, you will lose containment, converting the situation into uncontrolled venous hemorrhage. Very rapidly you will find yourself trying to squeeze the toothpaste back into the tube.

The correct approach is not to mobilize the liver and stay well away from the bare area. Instead, return to the chest and simply close the posterior diaphragmatic hole with a couple of big stitches. This simple solution will re-establish containment, keep Pandora's Box closed, and prevent the catastrophic hemorrhage.

Never open Pandora's Box!

THE KEY POINTS

▶ Five compartments converge in the thoracoabdominal region.

▶ Every bullet tells a story.

▶ Maintain tactical flexibility.

▶ Mobilize the left lateral lobe for transdiaphragmatic pericardiotomy.

▶ When fixing the diaphragm, pull it toward you.

▶ Never open Pandora's Box!

Chapter 11
The No-nonsense Trauma Thoracotomy

Life is pleasant. Death is peaceful.
It's the transition that's troublesome.

~ Isaac Asimov

Imagine playing a new computer game. The plot takes place in one or more of five domains or territories. While you're exploring one domain, the real action may well be unfolding in another. Each domain has a separate portal, and choosing the wrong portal for a specific game lands you in deep trouble from the get-go. To make things even more interesting, the game has a different storyline in each territory. To top everything, your game is fast-paced and short - with no replays.

Beginning to think that you don't want to play? Sorry, it's not a game, and you have no choice. It's thoracotomy for trauma, an operation that often starts as a good case and quickly turns into an operative roller coaster, especially if you are a general surgeon who does not frequently visit the chest. The action can unfold in one or more of five separate visceral compartments (two pleural spaces, pericardial space, thoracic outlet, and posterior mediastinum), each accessible through a different incision. Several pathophysiological mechanisms may be at work simultaneously: bleeding, hypoxia, cardiac tamponade, tension pneumothorax, and air embolism, each evolving at a different pace. Get the picture?

Where to cut?

Choosing the correct incision may well be your most important strategic decision in a trauma thoracotomy. The wrong incision can turn a straightforward case into a technical nightmare.

For the hemodynamically unstable patient in need of a crash operation, the utility incision is an anterolateral thoracotomy through the 4th intercostal space on the injured side. This quick incision keeps your options open. You can easily extend it across the sternum to the other side of the chest or go into the abdomen without having to reposition the patient. However, flexibility comes at a price. While an anterolateral thoracotomy allows you to get to all parts of the ipsilateral lung, trying to reach a deep posterior chest wall bleeder or a posterior mediastinal structure may be virtually impossible.

For a penetrating wound to the right lower chest with hemothorax, consider going into the abdomen first. The liver dominates the right thoracoabominal region and is, therefore, the most likely source of severe hemorrhage (Chapter 10).

> **Begin with anterolateral thoracotomy in the unstable patient**

Median sternotomy is a good incision for precordial stab wounds, since it gives you full access to the heart and great vessels of the upper mediastinum. Its biggest advantage is extensibility; you can easily carry it into the abdomen, neck, or along the clavicle. It also provides access to the hilum of each lung, but access to the periphery of the lung is restricted, and the posterior mediastinum is inaccessible.

In the patient actively bleeding from penetrating trauma to the thoracic outlet, you can stumble into a big trap if you choose the wrong incision. You must base your decision on an educated guess as to the source of hemorrhage. If the patient presents in shock with a large hemothorax, you typically begin with the utility anterolateral thoracotomy but may discover you cannot repair the injury through this incision. You must then rapidly extend it (or make a new one) to get to the bleeder.

If the patient is not actively bleeding into the pleural space, median sternotomy is a good incision for right-sided and midline thoracic outlet wounds, giving you access to the innominate artery and its branches. However, it is difficult to get to the left subclavian artery from the front because the vessel is intrapleural and posterior. So, in a patient with a penetrating injury above or below the left clavicle, gain proximal control of the subclavian artery through a high left anterolateral thoracotomy in the 3rd intercostal space (above the nipple), recognizing that you cannot fix the vessel through this very limited incision. You will have to expose the injured subclavian artery through a separate incision (Chapter 13).

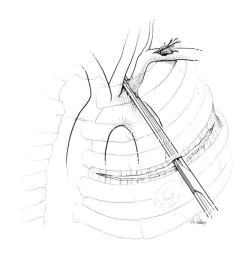

The classic trap door incision is a creative combination of a median sternotomy, left anterolateral thoracotomy, and a left clavicular incision. It requires forceful retraction to open the upper mediastinum and has a high incidence of postoperative causalgia-like pain due to stretching of the brachial plexus and other nerves. We never use it because you can achieve the same exposure using just two of the three elements of the trap door with much less morbidity.

Stable patients hide fewer surprises. You know your surgical target from preoperative imaging, and this target dictates your choice of incision. Extensibility into another visceral compartment is usually not a consideration. Posterior mediastinal structures such as the aorta or esophagus are approached through a posterolateral thoracotomy at a level corresponding to the injury. In fact, posterolateral thoracotomy provides such outstanding exposure of the chest wall, lung, and mediastinum that one of us occasionally uses it in actively bleeding patients, especially if the penetrating wound is posterior and low.

Carefully select your incision for thoracic outlet injury

Anterolateral thoracotomy made easy

Place the patient supine with both arms extended, and shove a rolled sheet behind the scapula to slightly lift and medially rotate the operated side of the chest. A double-lumen endotracheal tube rapidly placed by a competent anesthesiologist gives you a huge technical advantage. Working around a collapsed lung is a walk in the park compared with the torture of trying to squeeze your way around a rhythmically inflating balloon.

Make a bold cut in the 4th intercostal space. In a male patient, this is below the nipple. In a female, retract the breast cranially and make the incision in the inframammary fold. Avoid the bulk of the pectoralis major by placing the incision immediately below it.

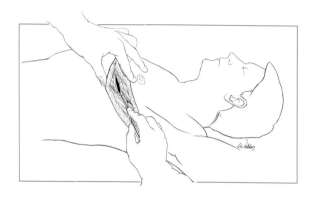

Think of this operation as the thoracic equivalent of a crash laparotomy. Work quickly and deliberately. This is not the time to be minimally invasive or go hunting for stray erythrocytes with your thunder stick. Just grab a knife and go into the chest. Carry your incision from the sternal border to the midaxillary line, following the intercostal space in a slight upward curve. Laterally, you soon encounter the law of diminishing returns: the further you extend your incision, the more muscle you have to cut with less exposure gained.

An experienced surgeon enters the chest with three bold strokes of the knife: the first divides the skin and subcutaneous tissue; the second cuts through the pectoralis fascia, the pectoralis muscle anteriorly and the serratus laterally; the third is a short incision in the intercostal muscles that brings you into the pleural space.

Grab a knife and dive into the chest

Once you have created a window into the pleural space, feel for any adhesions between the lung and the chest wall. If the way is clear, take a pair of heavy Mayo scissors and boldly cut the intercostal muscles along your line of incision. Insert a rib spreader into the incision with the handle toward the axilla; otherwise, the handle will be in your way when you try to extend the incision

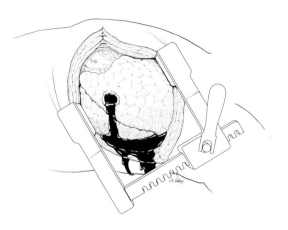

across the sternum. Open the rib spreader carefully to create your work space.

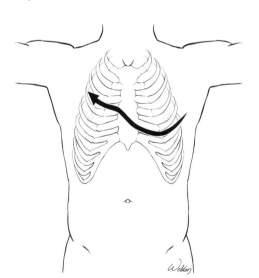

If necessary, extend your incision to the other side of the chest by cutting across the sternum cleanly using a Gigli saw, an oscillating saw, or bone cutters. When crossing the sternum from left to right, carry the incision upward to the 3rd intercostal space to stay above the right nipple, thus facilitating exposure of the upper mediastinal structures, especially the innominate bifurcation.

The classic pitfall in anterolateral thoracotomy is failure to identify and ligate the transected ends of the internal mammary artery. When the patient is hypotensive and vasoconstricted, this deceitful artery seldom bleeds. After you close the chest, it soon makes its presence known. If you don't tie the transected ends, you guarantee your patient an early return to the OR.

Don't forget the internal mammary artery because it won't forget you

---

Once inside the chest

In most trauma thoracotomies you will not have the benefit of a double-lumen tube, and the anesthesiologist will not be able to drop the lung upon request. With the lung inflated, you initially see little except a rhythmically bulging balloon and blood around it. To explore the chest, you must mobilize the lung.

The key maneuver is cutting the inferior pulmonary ligament. Gently place your non-dominant hand below the lower lobe of the lung, pull it cranially to put the inferior pulmonary ligament on tension, and divide it with scissors. Remember that the ligament ends at the inferior pulmonary vein, and a lacerated pulmonary vein 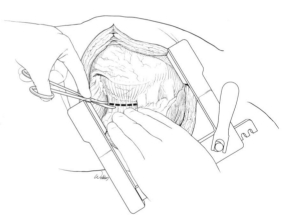 may bring your operation to a spectacular premature end. Now, you can retract the lung and work around it.

Mobilize the lung by cutting the inferior pulmonary ligament

Evacuate the blood, ask the anesthesiologist to stop inflating the lung for a moment, and rapidly assess the situation. Where is the bleeding coming from? Lung or chest wall? Do you suspect a pericardial tamponade? Is there a mediastinal hematoma? Bright red blood pooling in the chest is frequently from chest wall bleeders, whereas a mixture of blood and bubbles usually comes from the lung. Gushes of dark blood are the hallmark of a pulmonary hilar injury. Mediastinal hematoma indicates potential large vessel injury. A bulging tense pericardium is a tamponade until proven otherwise. Obtain temporary control of bleeding by packing the chest wall, manually compressing the pulmonary hilum of a massively bleeding lung, or opening the pericardium to release a tamponade. Once you have temporary control of hemorrhage, decide whether you are dealing with BIG TROUBLE or a small problem (Chapter 2).

Are you worried about the other side of the chest? You certainly should be because you cannot see it. Any doubts about bleeding in the other pleural space (e.g. suspicious trajectory or unexplained hypotension) should prompt you to push your hand immediately anterior to the pericardium to create a window into the other hemithorax. Is blood pouring out of your window? Can you scoop up blood and clots when you push your hand into the lateral recesses of the pleural space? If so, you must explore the other side.

Next, optimize your work space. Is your incision adequate or do you need better exposure? Using bone cutters, you can divide the costal cartilage of the 4th rib at the upper edge of your incision to allow the rib spreader to open wider. If time is critical, open the rib spreader as much as you have to, even if you feel a rib cracking. This is not an elective thoracotomy, and you must have adequate exposure, whatever it takes. If all this is still not enough, the ace up your sleeve is, of course, a clam-shell extension across the sternum that will expose everything. It is, however, an incision that carries significant morbidity.

You may wish to do something about the lung that is rhythmically billowing in your face. You can ask the anesthesiologist to reduce the tidal volume to enable you to work around the lung, or you can help push the endotracheal tube into the contralateral bronchus. This "mainstemming" is much easier on the right, although the right upper lobe may remain non-ventilated. On the left side, it is difficult to blindly push the tube into the mainstem bronchus. Exchanging an endotracheal tube for a double-lumen tube in mid-operation is difficult and dangerous. Consider it with much apprehension and only if nothing else works.

> **Optimize your work space and drop the lung if you can**

Opening the pericardium

A classic error of inexperience is leaving the pericardium unopened because it looks okay from the outside. With the pericardium, what you see is not what you get, and a normal appearing sac can easily hide a tamponade. During a left anterolateral thoracotomy, retract the left lung

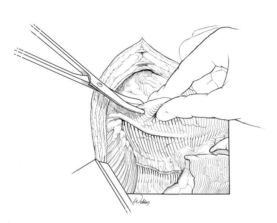

posteriorly to expose the left lateral aspect of the pericardium. Pinch it with your fingers to tent it up and make a nick with scissors anterior to the phrenic nerve. If you see blood draining through the hole, widely open the pericardium by sliding the slightly open scissors parallel to the phrenic nerve, and deliver the heart into the open chest.

If you find blood in the pericardial sac during a right anterolateral thoracotomy, immediately extend into a clam-shell incision. You cannot properly examine or fix the injured heart from the right side.

> **The closed pericardium is an enigma - open it!**

Controlling the pulmonary hilum

Massive bleeding from a central lung injury requires swift control of the hilum. Hilar clamping is a "doomsday weapon" because it is poorly tolerated by a patient in shock. If you can stop the bleeding by any other means, such as manual pressure, hemostatic suture, or rapid resection of the injured segment - don't clamp the hilum.

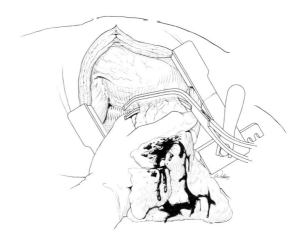

You can't even begin to encircle the hilum unless the lung is mobilized by cutting the inferior pulmonary ligament. Ask the anesthesiologist to stop ventilating the lungs momentarily, and gather the partially-inflated lung in your non-dominant hand like a bouquet of flowers. Negotiate a Satinsky clamp around the entire hilum, taking care to avoid injury to the phrenic nerve, which is alarmingly close. Pulmonary hilar clamping requires both hands; one hand holds the open clamp while the other guides the jaws around the hilum.

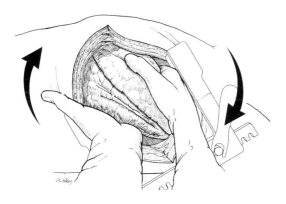

Clamping the hilum within the restricted work space provided by an anterolateral thoracotomy can be tricky because you often cannot see what you are doing. There is a simpler way to do it. You can twist the lung around the hilum - the pulmonary hilar twist. Instead of trying to negotiate an open clamp around the hilum, simply grab the mobilized lung with both hands, holding the apex of the upper lobe and base of the lower. Now, twist the lung 180° so that the apex of the upper lobe abuts the diaphragm and the base of the lung is now where the apex resided until a few seconds ago. Bleeding stops immediately. You may need to place a laparotomy pad in the upper pleural space to keep the lung in the upside-down position. This quick and simple maneuver is particularly useful during ER thoracotomy, where exposure and working conditions are severely compromised.

Twist the lung to rapidly control the hilum without a clamp

Aortic clamping

The descending thoracic aorta is flaccid and pulseless, easily mistaken for an adjacent flaccid pulseless tube, the esophagus. Clamping the esophagus does not improve the patient's hemodynamics one bit.

Placing a clamp on the descending thoracic aorta during an urgent anterolateral thoracotomy is guided mostly by palpation rather than direct vision. Retract the left lung anteriorly and slide your hand on the posterior chest wall from lateral to medial, feeling the concavity of the posterior ribs as they arch toward the spine. The first tubular structure you feel against the tip of your fingers is the aorta. You can either manually compress it against the spine or place an aortic clamp across it, freeing your hand for other useful work.

The key to succ-essful clamping is to open the parietal pleura. If the media-stinal pleura overlying the aorta remains intact, your clamp will slide off and without obtaining a purchase on the vessel.

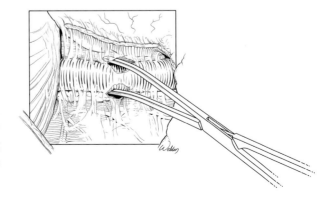

Make a hole in the parietal pleura on both sides of the aorta, either with your finger or Mayo scissors. All you need is a limited opening, just enough to accommodate a clamp, on each side of the flaccid tube. More extensive dissection may avulse an intercostal vessel or injure the aorta itself, making matters much worse.

You can't clamp the aorta over intact parietal pleura

The "turbo" version

The turbo version of a thoracotomy for trauma is the much-advertised ER (or resuscitative) thoracotomy, a heroic operation typically begun in the shock room but, if successful, always concluded in the OR. To begin a resuscitative thoracotomy, all you need is an endotracheal tube in place, a steady hand, a decent knife, and a brain in gear.

Fully abduct the patient's left arm to get it out of your way, have someone squirt iodine on the left chest, and start cutting. While sterility is not a central issue here, your safety is. Sharp instruments and needles are prominently in play during resuscitative thoracotomy. A cardinal rule, therefore, is to have only one pair of hands in the operative field - yours. Accidental sticks and cuts are a clear and present danger in the organized chaos of a resuscitative thoracotomy, and patients with penetrating trauma often carry transmissible diseases. Don't kill yourself or injure a colleague while trying to save your patient.

Resuscitative thoracotomy is a classic damage control procedure. After you open the chest, only five maneuvers are done in the ER.

The Five Moves of ER Thoracotomy

Incise the inferior pulmonary ligament to mobilize the lung
Open the pericardium and staple (or suture) a cardiac laceration
Perform open cardiac massage
Clamp the pulmonary hilum or twist a massively bleeding lung
Clamp the thoracic aorta

If the patient survives, do everything else in the OR. If organized electrical activity does not return within a reasonable period of time, recognize failure and stop. Don't endanger your team in futile situations. Regardless of your surgical talents and experience, you will not have many survivors of resuscitative thoracotomy.

Worry about personal and team safety in a resuscitative thoracotomy

---

Median sternotomy

Make a vertical incision in the sternal midline extending from 2cm above the sternal notch to 3-4cm below the xiphoid. Deepen your incision to the anterior table of the sternum, keeping to the midline. Define the superior border of the manubrium and bluntly develop the retrosternal plane from above with your finger. Then, go to the inferior part of your incision and open the linea alba immediately caudal to the xiphoid to bluntly develop the same plane from below.

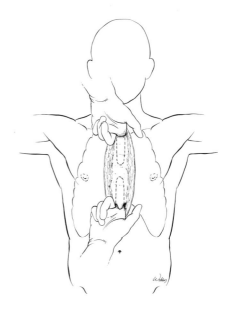

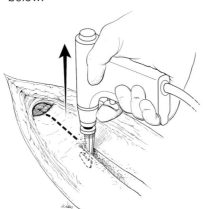

Ask the anesthesiologist to stop ventilating momentarily, divide the sternum in the midline using a vertical sternal saw. Hook the toe of the saw beneath the sternum and pull on it to elevate the bone as it is being cut to reduce the risk of iatrogenic injury to substernal structures. Use the cautery to control oozing from the cut edges of the bone. Insert a sternal

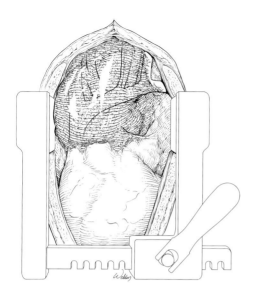

retractor and gradually open it without cracking the sternum.

What you are looking for is the left innominate vein, the gatekeeper of the thoracic outlet. Extending across the anterior aspect of the upper mediastinum, it is the first structure you have to deal with when dissecting in the thoracic outlet. In the trauma situation, identify, clamp, divide, and ligate the vein.

> **The left innominate vein is the gatekeeper of the upper mediastinum**

Closing the chest

Much like trauma laparotomy, you have to choose between definitive and temporary closure of the chest. In either case, place chest tubes in the operated pleural space or in the mediastinum and inspect the chest wall carefully for intercostal, muscular, and internal mammary bleeders.

When should you consider temporary closure? It is a valid option when you are racing against the patient's rapidly deteriorating physiology or when you intend to return to the chest to remove packs or perform definitive repairs. Temporary closure of the chest means approximating only the skin to achieve airtight closure, leaving the ribs and chest wall muscles unapproximated. You can rapidly close the skin edges with either a continuous heavy monofilament suture or a series of towel clips. Rarely, when the heart is swollen and edematous and will not allow even skin closure of a median sternotomy incision, we temporarily suture an empty intravenous fluid bag to the skin edges while the underlying sternum remains open. This is the thoracic equivalent of the plastic bag closure described in Chapter 4.

Skin-only closure of an anterolateral thoracotomy has one big drawback: it bleeds. While making the incision, you typically divide a substantial mass of chest wall muscles in the lateral part of the incision. If you don't approximate this muscle mass, you will have continuous oozing that may translate into significant ongoing blood loss, especially if the patient is coagulopathic.

Formal closure of an anterolateral thoracotomy is straightforward. Approximate the ribs using heavy pericostal sutures followed by layered closure of the chest wall muscles, fascia and skin. In closing a clam-shell incision, take special care to precisely reapproximate the divided sternum using sternal wires.

THE KEY POINTS

▶ Begin with anterolateral thoracotomy in the unstable patient.

▶ Carefully select your incision for thoracic outlet injury.

▶ Grab a knife and dive into the chest.

▶ Don't forget the internal mammary artery because it won't forget you.

▶ Mobilize the lung by cutting the inferior pulmonary ligament.

▶ Optimize your work space and drop the lung if you can.

▶ The closed pericardium is an enigma - open it!

▶ Twist the lung to rapidly control the hilum without a clamp.

▶ You can't clamp the aorta over intact parietal pleura.

▶ Worry about personal and team safety in a resuscitative thoracotomy.

▶ The left innominate vein is the gatekeeper of the upper mediastinum.

Chapter 12
The Chest: Inside and Out

Good judgment comes from experience.
Experience comes from poor judgment.

~ Arthur C. Beall, Jr., MD

You are inside the right chest doing a thoracotomy for a gunshot injury to the low posterior back. You are relieved to see the lung is not bleeding. Bright red blood is coming from the bullet hole in the chest wall, probably from an intercostal artery. It looks like a simple problem that just needs a hemostatic stitch. Then, as you try to get to the bleeder, deep down in the inaccessible recesses behind the diaphragm, it gradually dawns on you - things are far from simple.

With the lung rhythmically billowing in your face, you can barely see the bleeder. Even if you do, getting to it through an anterolateral thoracotomy is tough, sometimes impossible. When you finally get to it and try to insert a figure of 8 stitch, you discover you cannot take a good bite with the needle because you keep bumping into ribs. The intercostal space is just not wide enough to accommodate a full swing of the needle. Welcome to the big leagues!

You have just come across a notoriously underrated injury - one of the "hidden monsters" of trauma surgery. It is certainly not the only one around. There is, in fact, an entire zoo. An injury around the EG junction (Chapter 5), a bleeding hole in the psoas muscle (Chapter 9), and blunt trauma to the lower extremity vessels below the knee (Chapter 15) are good examples. They are not as dramatic as a shattered liver or a gunshot to the surgical soul and may seem straightforward at first glance. But when you take them on, you discover you are in deeper waters than you thought, sometimes well over your head. The hidden monsters of trauma tax your operative creativity and imagination, forcing you to come up with unorthodox solutions.

Bleeding from the chest wall

The intercostal and internal mammary arteries bleed furiously because they have a bidirectional blood supply. To achieve effective hemostasis, you must control the artery from both sides. The challenging chest wall bleeder is not the one located immediately beneath your incision staring you in the face when you open the chest. It is the cunning, unreachable injury, very high or very low on the chest wall - a bleeder you can barely see.

Your first priority is temporary control. Rapidly assess the situation: can you see the spurting vessel? Are you dealing with a discrete artery (in penetrating trauma) or with diffuse oozing from extensive trauma to chest wall muscles (in blunt trauma)? Are the adjacent ribs fractured? Is there more than one source of bleeding? Depending on your findings, compress the bleeder with your finger, clamp it, or temporarily pack it.

Next, optimize your exposure. If the bleeder is very low or very high on the chest wall, you may have to make a new lower (or higher) incision to get to it. A neat trick is to move two intercostal spaces up or down through the *same* skin incision and re-enter the chest through a more appropriate intercostal space, giving yourself a better shot at controlling the injury. In some cases you may need a new skin incision.

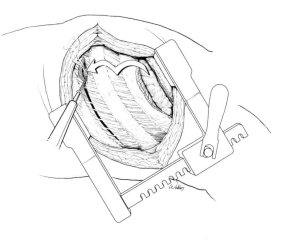

Now, choose an appropriate hemostatic technique. If the bleeding vessel is right in front of you, simply clamp and suture-ligate it. This is usually possible with the internal mammary artery because it runs perpendicular to the ribs and is relatively easy to reach in its anterior location. A transected intercostal artery is more challenging. It often retracts in between the surrounding intercostal muscles and requires a blind hemostatic figure of 8 suture.

The secret of success is not only choosing the correct needle size, but also orienting the needle path to be parallel - not perpendicular - to the adjacent ribs. There is not enough space between the ribs to accommodate a full perpendicular swing of a large needle, so unless you drive the needle parallel to the ribs you won't be able to complete the arc and extract it.

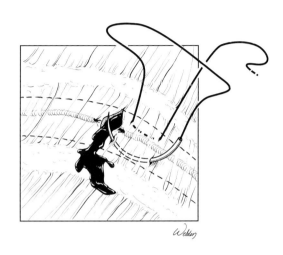

What should you do if the hemostatic stitch doesn't work? Here, a little tactical creativity can go a long way. Consider using hemostatic metal clips. Alternatively, if the immediately adjacent rib is shattered into several fragments, rapidly resecting a fragment adjacent to the bleeding vessel can give you valuable space for maneuvering.

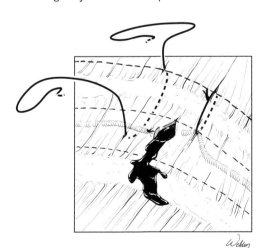

If all else fails, take a heavy monofilament suture on a large needle and encircle the entire rib immediately cephalad to the bleeding intercostal vessel, ligating the neurovascular bundle *on masse* and compressing it against the rib. Do it both proximal and distal to the bleeding site. Postoperative intercostal neuralgia is an acceptable price for this lifesaving maneuver.

Another last resort technique that works with large bleeding craters from high caliber gunshots is balloon tamponade. Insert a large Foley balloon catheter through the missile tract from outside into the chest, inflate the balloon, and pull hard to tamponade the bleeding. Clamp the Foley flush with the chest wall to maintain traction on the catheter, and suture the clamp to the skin to prevent accidental dislodgment. Leave this compressing balloon in place for a few days to ensure thrombosis of the injured artery. We have also stuffed bleeding bullet tracts in the deep posterior chest wall with local hemostatic agents or bone wax, much like we do with the hosing vertebral artery in the neck (Chapter 14).

A most frustrating situation is diffuse multifocal oozing from extensive damage to the chest wall, with multiple associated rib fractures. Direct hemostasis doesn't work, and you rapidly realize your only option is to control obvious arterial bleeders, pack the damaged chest wall, and rapidly bail out. These are often lethal injuries.

Suture intercostal bleeders parallel to the ribs

The injured lung

Despite obvious anatomical differences, the bleeding lung is strikingly similar to the injured liver. In both organs, you deal with peripheral injuries using a variety of hemostatic techniques, while central injuries (close to the hilum) are very bad news. In both lung and liver, surgeons use hilar control and non-anatomical segmental resection but are wary of formal extensive resection (lobectomy in the liver, pneumonectomy in the lung). The concept of tractotomy, a most useful technique for through-and-through lung injuries, was originally borrowed from hepatic trauma.

You can suture superficial pulmonary lacerations, but your most effective weapon in dealing with the bleeding lung is *stapled non-anatomic resection.* How is it done?

Define the precise location of the injury and use a linear cutting stapler to rapidly open the interlobar fissure, if fused. Now, take a good look at the injured lung segment and plan your line of resection. Your aim is to remove the injured tissue with the least amount of surrounding healthy parenchyma. Have all staplers and 3:0 or 4:0 poplypropylene sutures

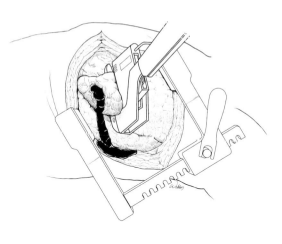

readily available before you start. Ask the anesthesiologist to momentarily deflate the injured lung. Use either a wide linear stapler (60 or 90mm) or several applications of a linear cutting stapler to resect the injured parenchyma. If the stapled line of resection continues to ooze or leak air, underrun it with a continuous monofilament suture.

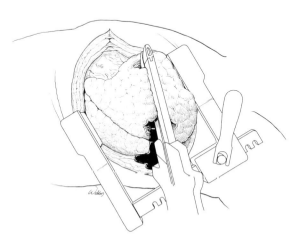

Pulmonary tractotomy is a an elegant lung-sparing solution for through-and-through penetrating injuries that are too deep for a stapled resection. The underlying principle is to lay open the tract so you can get to the bleeders inside it. In other words, you connect the tract to the lung surface by dividing the bridge of tissue between them.

Insert one arm of a linear cutting stapler (we prefer to use a vascular staple load) into the missile tract and apply the other arm to your chosen target surface. Close the stapler and fire it, laying the missile tract wide open. Now, carefully inspect it for bleeding vessels and suture-ligate them selectively using 4:0 polypropylene. Do not close the tract.

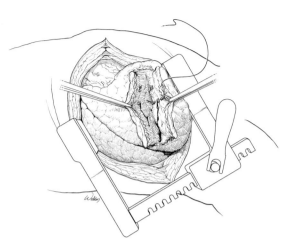

If you don't have a linear cutting stapler, you can do the same tractotomy between two long aortic clamps applied to the bridge of tissue overlying the missile tract. After selectively controlling bleeders in the open tract, underrun each aortic clamp with a 4:0 polypropylene suture before removing it.

Pulmonary tractotomy works so well that you should consider using it even in deep penetrating wounds that are not through-and-through (i.e. no exit wound). Insert a finger into the missile tract and assess how much uninjured lung parenchyma must be crossed to complete a through-and-through tract. If the distance is short, use the stapler as a "missile" to complete the tract, pushing it through the tract until the tip emerges from the other side of the lung. Part of the tract will be iatrogenic, but a tract is a tract, and therefore amenable to tractotomy. Lay it open and suture-ligate individual bleeders.

Pulmonary tractotomy is a neat solution to a difficult problem

---

BIG TROUBLE with the lung

Central lung injuries are deadly because they are difficult to control and repair. They are classic examples of **BIG TROUBLE** (Chapter 2), where organizing your attack and your team before jumping in can make an enormous difference.

When confronted with massive bleeding from an injury close to the pulmonary hilum, rapidly mobilize the lung, gathering it in your non-dominant hand, and pinch the bleeding hilum between thumb and forefinger. The similarity to the Pringle maneuver is obvious. Now organize your attack: improve exposure, "mainstem" the

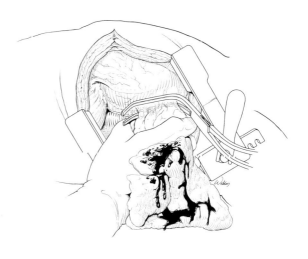

endotracheal tube into the contralateral bronchus if possible, and get a full set of vascular instruments and an autotransfusion device.

At this point, your options depend primarily on the mechanism of injury. With a simple stab wound, pinching the injured hilum may give you just enough control and visibility to rapidly do a lateral repair using 5:0 polypropylene. The situation bears an uncanny resemblance to the injured portal vein in the hepatoduodenal ligament. In both cases, you are dealing with a lacerated low-pressure (but high-flow) system within a very narrow anatomic space that affords you little room for maneuvering or comfortable clamping.

> **Control the pulmonary hilum between thumb and forefinger**

A central gunshot injury is bad news. Damage is more extensive, you often must clamp the hilum, and may be forced to resect a lobe (or even the entire lung) to achieve hemostasis. A theorctically appealing option for hilar injuries is vascular control from within the pericardium because it is based on the principle of anatomical barriers (Chapter 3).

If you open the pericardium anterior and parallel to the phrenic nerve, you are working in uninjured virgin territory, much like working above the inguinal ligament in a groin gunshot wound. However, this takes time and requires thorough knowledge of intrapericardial anatomy - not a good option for the general trauma surgeon facing a central lung injury in a rapidly exsanguinating patient. In practice, a gunshot wound close to the pulmonary hilum means a rapid lobectomy or, in extreme circumstances, pneumonectomy.

A stapled pneumonectomy is a technically simple but physiologically devastating operative maneuver, so use it as an absolute last resort. Exsanguinating trauma patients do not tolerate acute removal of the lung. Pneumonectomy stops the bleeding but often leads to acute right heart failure, hemodynamic collapse, and very high mortality.

If, despite all efforts, you have no choice but to take out the lung, bring a 90mm linear stapler with a vascular staple load across the entire hilum. The technical principle is to move the stapler as distal as possible to give yourself room for a suture line should stapling require reinforcement. Carefully close the stapler across the entire hilum, fire it, and remove the lung. Take hold of both edges of the stapled stump with Allis clamps, and only then release the stapler. There is always residual bleeding from the stapled line of resection. Control it with a running monofilament suture.

> **Do a stapled pneumonectomy only as a last resort**

The thoracic esophagus

Approach an injury to the upper and midthoracic esophagus through a right posterolateral thoracotomy in the 4th intercostal space. The injured lower thoracic esophagus is accessed through a left posterolateral thoracotomy in the 6-7th intercostal space.

The bail out solution for an esophageal perforation is proximal drainage to convert the free perforation into a controlled fistula. The cardinal sin is creating a dead-end esophageal pouch above the injury, an undrained "pus sausage" that is a source of ongoing sepsis and slowly kills the patient.

Drain the perforation by inserting a large-bore suction drain through the perforation and up into the proximal esophagus, and secure it in place. If you can get an esophageal T-tube, use it. If possible, approximate the edges of the hole around the drain. Always remember to drain the pleural space with a separate drain or a tube thoracostomy. Use this damage control option

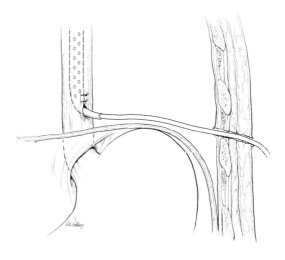

when you have to bail out in a hurry, the injury is too large to be approximated without tension, or the operation is delayed (more than 12-24 hours from injury) and the pleural space is severely inflamed, making primary closure unsafe.

An esophageal perforation is a hole in the gut. If you decide to close it, always begin by carefully debriding and defining the edges of the mucosal defect, just as you would do for any other part of the GI tract. Do not mobilize the esophagus out of its bed because you will devascularize it, jeopardizing your repair. Close the perforation in two layers (mucosa and muscle), and drain the pleural space.

Cover the repair with a vascularized pedicle of tissue. Depending on the operative circumstances, this can be an intercostal muscle flap, a Thal patch of gastric fundus (Chapter 5), or a chunk of omentum. Pericardial or pleural flaps are not well-vascularized in the acute setting, so don't use them. Provide a route for early enteral feeding.

Drain an esophageal perforation as a bail out solution

The major airways

The close anatomical proximity of the major airways to the great vessels, esophagus, and lungs virtually guarantees you will rarely encounter an isolated injury to the intrathoracic trachea or a major bronchus. Major airway injury typically takes second seat to hemorrhage because gushing blood takes priority over leaking air.

The damage control solution for an intrathoracic tracheal injury is to negotiate the endotracheal tube past the injury, bypassing it to prevent a massive air leak. For a mainstem bronchus injury, the bail out solution is mainstemming the endotracheal tube into the contralateral bronchus (Chapter 11). Air leaks from smaller airways can be managed initially with a chest tube, with delayed resection of the involved lobe.

If, during thoracotomy for trauma, you encounter a straightforward laceration of the trachea or a major bronchus, fix it with a single row of interrupted absorbable sutures. Do not use a non-absorbable suture in the airways; it leads to granuloma formation and later stenosis. For all other injuries that require complex reconstructions, the smartest thing you can do is resist the temptation to tackle them on your own, and get the help of an experienced thoracic surgeon.

Fix straightforward major airway injuries with absorbable suture

---

THE KEY POINTS

▶   Suture intercostal bleeders parallel to the ribs.

▶   Pulmonary tractotomy is a neat solution to a difficult problem.

▶   Control the pulmonary hilum between thumb and forefinger.

▶   Do a stapled pneumonectomy only as a last resort.

▶   Drain an esophageal perforation as a bail out solution.

▶   Fix straightforward major airway injuries with absorbable suture.

Chapter 13
Thoracic Vascular Trauma for the General Surgeon

The road to the heart is only 2-3cm in a direct line, but it has taken surgery nearly 2400 years to travel it.

~ H.M. Sherman

Injuries to the heart and thoracic great vessels have an irritating tendency to force themselves on you. If you are a general surgeon, the major vascular structures of the chest are not your natural habitat, and you would much rather have a cardiothoracic colleague deal with them. With blunt aortic injuries this is not only possible but is also a good idea because you are dealing with a contained hematoma. There is time to delineate the injury by angiography, consider various options (including endovascular repair), or transfer the patient to another facility. Not so with penetrating trauma, where the patient is actively bleeding and often in shock. You must take a deep breath - and plunge in. A phone call to a cardiac surgeon is not a valid resuscitative maneuver for cardiac tamponade.

This chapter deals with thoracic cardiovascular trauma from the perspective of the general surgeon. Most penetrating injuries to the heart and thoracic great vessels can be fixed using straightforward vascular principles and techniques. If you gain rapid access to the injury and keep your wits about you, you have a good chance of saving the patient.

Accessing the bleeding heart

The operative encounter with a stabbed heart is often one of the most rewarding experiences a surgical resident can have. It involves a rapid simple procedure that revives a patient who, until a few minutes earlier, was virtually dead. Don't let this gratifying experience mislead you. Cardiac injuries can also be extremely vicious and lethal. They come in two flavors: simple and complex.

A simple cardiac injury is a small accessible laceration, most often a stab wound. Outcome is determined by how quickly you crack the chest and release the tamponade. These patients don't die of exsanguination, and cardiac repair is usually easy.

Complex injuries are multiple, inaccessible, large, or involve the coronary arteries. Release of tamponade is only the first step in an uphill battle. Complex cardiac wounds are BIG TROUBLE (Chapter 2), carrying very high mortality rates even in the most experienced hands.

How do you get to the wounded heart? If you have already begun with a resuscitative thoracotomy, open the pericardium longitudinally, anterior to the phrenic nerve. Release the tamponade and deliver the heart into the operative field. Injuries to the right side of the right ventricle or to the right atrium cannot be reached through a left anterolateral thoracotomy, so extend your incision across the sternum.

If the patient is not *in extremis*, consider doing a median sternotomy. This incision takes a little more time, and your access to a posterior cardiac wound from the front is more difficult. We prefer a left anterolateral thoracotomy for most cardiac wounds, especially gunshot injuries that often involve damage to other thoracic structures. We reserve median sternotomy for precordial stab wounds in relatively stable patients.

> **Do a left anterolateral thoracotomy for cardiac gunshot wounds**

Temporary bleeding control

Once inside the pericardium, rapidly evacuate blood and clots, locate the injury, and select an appropriate temporary hemostatic technique. Your assistant's finger is an excellent first choice, but there are other options.

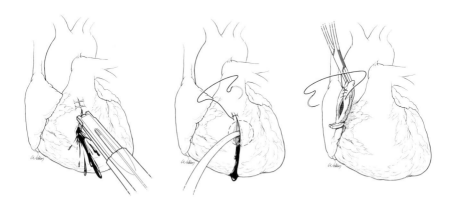

During resuscitative thoracotomy in the shock room, temporarily stapling the laceration with a skin stapler is a cool trick since a stapler is so much safer than a needle. Control a larger wound by inserting a Foley catheter through the hole and inflating it. Use a Satinsky side-biting clamp to control a right atrial laceration.

If the damage is extensive or the injury inaccessible, you may have to resort to temporary inflow occlusion. If you clamp both the superior and inferior venae cavae, the heart will empty and stop, giving you a couple of minutes (not more!) to suture the laceration in a dry field. If you are not a cardiac surgeon, the simplest way to achieve inflow occlusion is by compressing the right atrium manually against the heart in a lateral-to-medial direction so the atrium

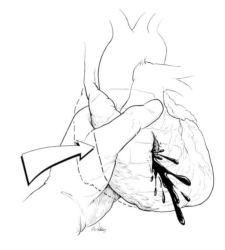

cannot fill. Use inflow occlusion only if you have no other choice. It is easy to stop the heart, but much more difficult to get it going again. In a cold, fibrillating heart, inflow occlusion will be a terminal event.

> **Inflow occlusion is your ultimate weapon in cardiac trauma**

Restarting the heart

When the heart is not contracting effectively, begin open cardiac compressions. If operating through a median sternotomy, compress the heart between both palms (without thumbs). In a left anterolateral thoracotomy your work space is limited, so compress with one hand against the sternum. Restart the heart using a combination of open cardiac massage, cross-clamping of the descending thoracic aorta, epinephrine (1mg) to achieve coarse ventricular fibrillation, and cardioversion using internal paddles applied directly to the heart at 10-30 Joules.

What should be your first priority if the bleeding heart is not contracting effectively? Should you fix the laceration first? Rapidly closing a cardiac laceration before it resumes dancing in front of you is certainly tempting, but it may take time, and your repair may fall apart when you compress the heart and inject inotropes. Epinephrine is the enemy of the myocardial suture line because it induces forceful contractions causing sutures to rip through the muscle. If you fix the laceration and then restart the heart, you may have to reinforce (or even redo) your suture line once the heart begins beating again.

Restarting the heart after repair may not be easy. A severely acidotic patient will benefit from a bolus of sodium bicarbonate prior to defibrillation. Even more important is external irrigation with warm saline to rewarm the heart immediately before applying the paddles. Use inotropes only if nothing else works.

> **Epinephrine is the enemy of the myocardial suture line**

Repairing simple cardiac wounds

Close a simple laceration with a 4:0 non-absorbable monofilament suture. Sewing the contracting myocardium is more difficult than optimistic illustrations like this lead you to believe. Not only are you working on a moving target, you also are dealing with a muscle that tears quite easily.

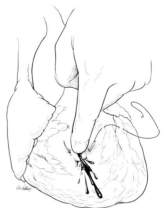

Some surgeons use Teflon pledgets to reinforce the suture line. We repair a lacerated ventricle with interrupted simple sutures. Your bites into the heart muscle should be deep but not full-thickness. The difficult part is not placing the sutures, but tying them. Unless you take special care not to tighten the knots too much, you will end up with a torn myocardium and a bigger hole to fix.

In an elderly patient or an edematous or friable myocardium, use horizontal mattress sutures with pledgets. Partial inflow occlusion by manually compressing the right atrium lowers pressures in the ventricles, a useful adjunct when sewing a compromised myocardium.

Since pressure in the right atrium is low, you often can control an atrial laceration temporarily with a partially occluding Satinsky-type clamp and then fix it with a running suture, as you would a large vein. Grazing non-penetrating myocardial wounds often bleed persistently and require suture repair just like a full-thickness laceration.

Tying sutures is the challenge when sewing heart wounds

Complex cardiac wounds

When you can't fix the injured heart with a few simple stitches, you are facing a bad situation, and your patient has a high likelihood of not making it. One such example is a posterior cardiac wound. To get to a posterior hole, you must lift the heart out of its bed, but the heart often protests by developing ventricular arrhythmia or arresting. In fact, tilting the heart up is another way of achieving inflow occlusion. Be aware of this when you manipulate the heart, and lift it gently and intermittently when addressing a posterior hole.

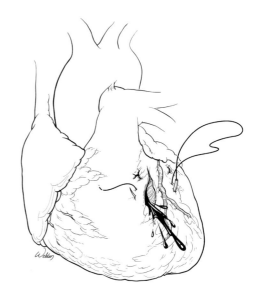

The technical solution for a laceration close to a coronary artery is a deep horizontal mattress suture that dives beneath the artery. Take special care when tying this suture because S-T segment changes or new Q waves on the ECG monitor may force you to remove the stitch and redo it. An injury to the coronary artery itself is typically distal since patients with transection of a proximal coronary vessel are usually dead on arrival. Your realistic option for a cardiac laceration with a transected distal coronary artery is to ligate the vessel and repair the hole, accepting the inevitable ischemia of the corresponding myocardial segment.

Cardiac tamponade caused by injury to the intrapericardial great vessels is usually lethal. On the rare occasion that you encounter it in a live patient, success hinges on your ability to rapidly identify the injury, temporarily control it with your finger or a Satinsky clamp, and fix it with simple lateral repair - much easier said than done.

In trauma atlases and textbooks you often see descriptions of heroic repair techniques for an injured coronary artery, patch repair of a large myocardial defect, or complex reconstructions of the intrapericardial great vessels. All these may be possible in special circumstances when a cardiothoracic surgeon and a pump team happen to be readily available. However, for the routine trauma patient arriving in the middle of the night with a penetrating cardiac injury and operated on by the trauma surgeon on call, they are science fiction.

Use quick and simple solutions for complex cardiac injuries

The thoracic outlet

How to explore a mediastinal hematoma

Median sternotomy provides excellent access to the superior mediastinum. A mediastinal hematoma looks like a large chunk of red jelly sitting above the pericardium, oozing blood and obscuring the anatomy. This red jelly usually signifies a major vascular injury in the thoracic outlet that you must find and fix.

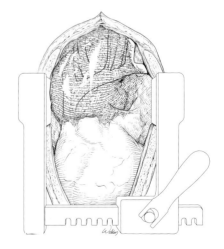

Exploring the superior mediastinum is remarkably similar to exploring the neck, as described in the next chapter. Both are essentially a trip through a minefield under sniper fire. You must follow a *trail of safety* from one key anatomical landmark to the next to guarantee a safe dissection and stay out of trouble.

Once inside the chest, identify the upper border of the pericardium. If the thymus is in your way, divide it between clamps and ligate it. You are looking for the left innominate vein. It is the gatekeeper of the mediastinum, just as the facial vein is in the neck. Dividing and ligating the left innominate vein opens up the superior mediastinum and gives you access to the superior aspect of the aortic arch and its branches.

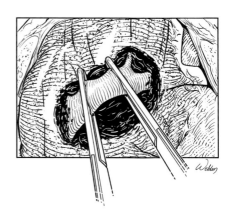

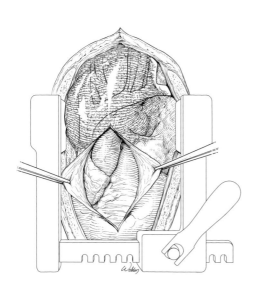

Dissection in a mediastinal hematoma is never easy. If you feel lost, a useful trick is to open the pericardium to orient yourself. The pericardium is an anatomical barrier that blocks the extension of the mediastinal hematoma, just like the inguinal ligament blocks the extension of a groin hematoma (Chapter 3). By opening the pericardium, you can follow the aortic arch upward into the hematoma to identify the vessels of the thoracic outlet.

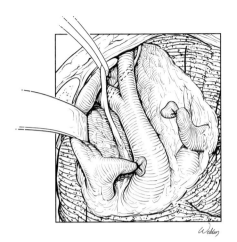

After identifying and dividing the left innominate vein, your next stop on the mediastinal trail of safety is the bifurcation of the innominate artery, the mediastinal equivalent of the carotid bifurcation in the neck. Your key landmark is the right vagus nerve as it crosses in front of the proximal right subclavian artery. Failure to identify the vagus in the mediastinum has the same consequences as it does in the neck - an invitation for iatrogenic injury.

Follow a trail of safety in exploring an upper mediastinal hematoma

---

Your next priority is proximal and distal control of the bleeding vessel. The vessels of the superior mediastinum are nicely arranged in two layers: superficial veins and deep arteries. Again, the similarities to the neck are striking. Control a venous injury with a side-biting clamp, and fix the hole. If a simple lateral repair will not do - ligate the vein without a second thought.

When dissecting the proximal left carotid artery, you must identify and preserve the left vagus nerve as it descends between the carotid and left subclavian arteries to cross in front of the aortic arch and give off the left recurrent laryngeal nerve. Proximal control of the left subclavian artery is discussed later in this chapter.

Never just plunge into a mediastinal hematoma from blunt trauma. The most common blunt arterial injury in the upper mediastinum is an innominate artery injury that presents as a contained hematoma (widened superior mediastinum) in a hemodynamically stable patient. Blindly entering the hematoma is the worst possible error you can make. The injury is avulsion of the take-off of the innominate artery from the aortic arch. In other words, you are dealing with a side-hole in the aorta. It doesn't take much surgical imagination to realize what will happen if you delve into this hematoma unprepared. The correct approach is briefly outlined in the next section of this chapter.

How about distal control of thoracic outlet injuries? As a general rule, the exposure provided by a median sternotomy is often not sufficient to allow distal control of the carotid and subclavian vessels. A median sternotomy is, however, an eminently extensile incision, so you can easily carry it into the neck or along the clavicle. If you are going into the neck, divide the strap muscles down low, near their insertion into the sternum, to expose the carotid sheath.

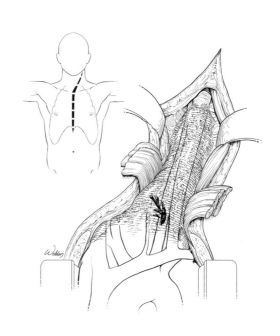

Never plunge blindly into the mediastinum in blunt trauma

Definitive repair and damage control options

In the upper mediastinum you almost never deal with an isolated penetrating injury to a single vessel. There are always associated injuries, and clamping the innominate or carotid artery carries a substantial risk of stroke. So don't fiddle with thoracic outlet injuries; use the simplest and quickest solution that will give an acceptable result. In most cases, this means a synthetic interposition graft. We prefer knitted Dacron rather than ePTFE because it is a softer graft with less needle-hole bleeding. The normal arteries of the thoracic outlet are extremely friable, and sewing them often feels like sewing wet tissue paper.

There are only limited damage control options in the thoracic outlet. Ligation of the injured artery is certainly an option if you accept the risk of stroke. A temporary intraluminal shunt is theoretically appealing and has been used twice by one of our colleagues but with no long-term survivors.

The only special vascular technique in the thoracic outlet is the "bypass and exclusion" repair of blunt innominate artery injury. If you aren't a cardiothoracic surgeon, you are unlikely to find yourself operating on this injury, since the patients are hemodynamically stable with a contained hematoma. You should, however, be familiar with the technical principle.

The bypass and exclusion repair begins by exposing the ascending aorta inside the pericardium and then obtaining distal control on the distal innominate, right subclavian and right carotid arteries. The surgeon deliberately avoids entering the hematoma around the proximal innominate artery. A partially occluding Satinsky clamp placed on the ascending aorta allows the surgeon to sew a 12mm knitted Dacron graft end-to-side to this side-clamped aortic segment. The innominate artery is then divided just proximal to its bifurcation, and the distal anastomosis (to the distal innominate) is completed. Only then is a second partially occluding clamp placed on the aorta around the take-off of the innominate artery. The hematoma is entered, and the side-hole in the excluded segment of aortic arch is closed with pledgeted sutures.

Use Dacron for thoracic outlet arterial reconstructions

The azygos vein

In penetrating chest trauma, azygos vein injury is seen in conjunction with injuries to the adjacent central airways, esophagus, or thoracic outlet vessels. The challenge with an azygos vein injury is getting to it. Access through a median sternotomy is extremely difficult, and it may even be difficult to reach through a right anterolateral thoracotomy, requiring an extension across the sternum. The injury is tough to identify because what you usually see is just a hole in the right posterior mediastinum hosing venous blood. Once identified, clamp and suture-ligate the injured vein, and meticulously search for associated injuries to the adjacent bronchus or esophagus.

The subclavian vessels

Before you embark on an adventure around the subclavian vessels, pause to assess how necessary it really is. Are you operating for bleeding or ischemia? If your circumstances are unfavorable (i.e. austere environment, lack of experience, other grave injuries), you may well be able to postpone the operation. If bleeding is from a missile tract, insert a Foley into it and inflate the balloon (Chapter 2). If this stops the bleeding, an immediate operation may not be necessary. If the arm is ischemic, a simple forearm fasciotomy can buy you valuable time. Endovascular stents or stent-grafts are effective alternatives to surgical repair of subclavian injuries in non-bleeding patients.

If you decide to proceed with an operation, proper positioning and draping are crucial. Place a shoulder roll vertically along the thoracic spine to drop the shoulders back. Support the head and rotate it to the contralateral side to extend the neck. Prep and drape the patient's chest with the upper extremity prepped free so it can initially be fully adducted at the patient's side and later abducted as necessary. You can get to the subclavian vessels through either a supraclavicular incision or the bed of the clavicle. Your choice of incision depends on the operative circumstances and your experience.

If you are not sure where the injury is located along the subclavian artery or if you don't have experience with subclavian exposure, the safest way to obtain proximal control is through the chest. Use a high (3rd interspace) left anterolateral thoracotomy incision for injury to the left subclavian artery, or median sternotomy if the injury is on the right.

When exploring a non-bleeding subclavian injury with minimal or no hematoma around the clavicle, we prefer a supraclavicular incision. Make your incision a fingerbreath above and parallel to the clavicle, extending from the sternal notch laterally to the distal third of the bone, a distance of approximately 8-10cm. Divide the platysma and place a self-retaining retractor in the wound. You must now go through two layers of muscle.

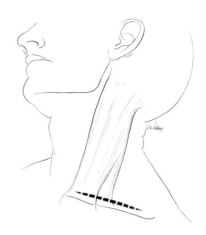

The first layer consists of the clavicular head of the sternocleidomastoid and the omohyoid laterally. Cut both muscles as close to the clavicle as possible, then reposition your retractor in a deeper plane to open the wound. If you see the internal jugular vein, define its lateral border and retract it medially out of harm's way. Now you can access and isolate the subclavian vein, but the artery is hiding one layer deeper down, behind the anterior scalene muscle.

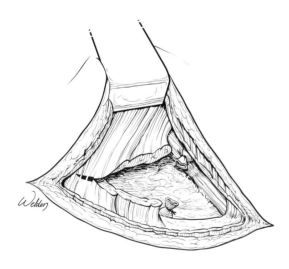

Behind the divided sternocleidomastoid, identify the scalene fat pad and carefully mobilize it from lateral to medial in search of the phrenic nerve. On the left side, you should be able to identify the thoracic duct as it enters the junction of the left subclavian and internal jugular veins. If injured, suture-ligate it with a 6:0 polypropylene suture; if not - leave it alone.

The key anatomical landmark in exposing the subclavian artery is the phrenic nerve behind the fat pad. During a subclavian exposure, it is the *only* structure you must preserve at any cost, even if the anatomy is hostile. It crosses the anterior scalene muscle from up and lateral to down and medial. Isolate the nerve on a vessel loop and gently retract it out of

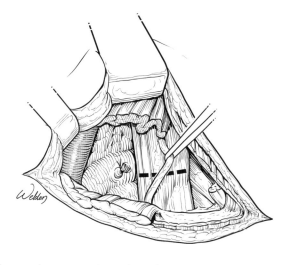

your way. Now cut the anterior scalene muscle as low down as you can. We divide the muscle piecemeal with scissors and not diathermy because it does not bleed and is close to the brachial plexus.

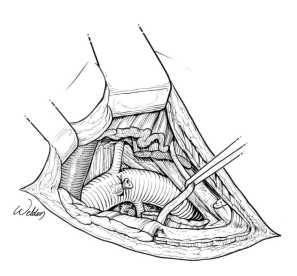

Only a thin periarterial fascia remains between you and the subclavian artery. Incise it to identify the periadventitial plane of safety and encircle the artery. The thyrocervical trunk is coming straight at you and is typically in your way. Dividing and ligating it helps you mobilize the subclavian artery. Clearly identify the vertebral and internal mammary arteries coming off the first part of the vessel to prevent accidental injury.

The phrenic nerve is your key to the subclavian artery

As always, things become considerably livelier when the subclavian artery is bleeding. An expanding hematoma fills the clavicular fossa, making it difficult to even palpate the clavicle. When operating under such adverse circumstances, we prefer to go through the bed of the clavicle because it's a quicker and simpler route.

Make your incision directly on the clavicle to expose the medial two-thirds of the bone. Score a line on the anterior surface of the bone with the diathermy. Now use a periosteal elevator to peel the periosteum off the clavicle in a circumferential fashion. Divide the clavicle as far laterally as you can with bone cutters or a saw, then grasp the medial fragment with a towel clip, and yank it out of its bed. Using the diathermy, take the head of the clavicle off the sternum. Cutting the subclavius muscle immediately deep to the clavicle brings you face-to-face with the pre-scalene fat pad and the phrenic nerve, and you know your way to the artery from there.

Distal control of the subclavian artery may require clamping the proximal axillary artery. If the clavicle is intact, clamp the axillary artery through a separate infraclavicular incision. However, if you removed the clavicle, you have an extensile incision that can be carried laterally toward the deltopectoral groove to expose the axillary artery.

The damage control options for an injured subclavian artery are ligation or temporary shunting. Both work. Ligation is usually well tolerated if the injury has not destroyed the major collateral pathways around the shoulder. Adding a pre-emptive forearm fasciotomy is a prudent move.

If you know your way around the injured subclavian artery and don't have to bail out, repair it. Unless dealing with a laceration that can be fixed with simple lateral repair, we again advise you go directly for an interposition graft. Mobilizing the soft and friable subclavian artery to gain enough length for an end-to-end repair almost never works. We isolate the injured segment and clamp it, define the injury, do a proximal and distal Fogarty thrombectomy, and insert an 8mm Dacron interposition graft. We do not replace the clavicle after completing the vascular reconstruction, but cover the repair with healthy muscle and soft tissue.

> **Go through the bed of the clavicle if the patient is bleeding**

The descending thoracic aorta

The patient with blunt injury to the descending thoracic aorta is typically hemodynamically stable and has a contained mediastinal hematoma. Don't forget that if the patient is unstable, the source of hemorrhage is almost invariably in *another* anatomical compartment, typically below the diaphragm.

Again, if you are not a cardiothoracic surgeon, you are not likely to find yourself in the left chest, face-to-face with a blunt aortic injury. However, be familiar with the general technical principles of the repair. Endovascular treatment offers an effective alternative to operative repair of these injuries. Although still under evaluation, this modality may become the preferred approach within the next few years.

The classic blunt aortic injury, located immediately distal to the take-off of the left subclavian artery, is repaired through a left posterolateral thoracotomy in the 4th intercostal space with single lung ventilation. The major pathophysiological challenge is central hypertension caused by proximal aortic clamping. Pharmacological agents, a passive shunt, or pump-assisted atriofemoral bypass, typically using a centrifugal pump and no heparin, are your options.

The technical difficulty in this operation stems from the close proximity of the aortic tear to the origin of the subclavian artery. The pleura overlying the proximal left subclavian artery is opened, and the artery is encircled by blunt dissection. Using a combination of sharp and blunt dissection, the surgeon then encircles the aorta between the left subclavian and left carotid arteries, creating just enough space to accommodate a clamp. The key maneuver is developing a plane between the undersurface of the aortic arch and the pulmonary artery. Distal control is obtained by encircling the distal thoracic aorta above the diaphragm.

After clamping, the hematoma is entered and a careful longitudinal aortotomy allows the surgeon to assess the extent of the injury and decide between primary repair (feasible in roughly 15% of cases) and Dacron graft interposition.

THE KEY POINTS

▶   Do a left anterolateral thoracotomy for cardiac gunshot wounds.

▶   Inflow occlusion is your ultimate weapon in cardiac trauma.

▶   Epinephrine is the enemy of the myocardial suture line.

▶   Tying sutures is the challenge when sewing heart wounds.

▶   Use quick and simple solutions for complex cardiac injuries.

▶   Follow a trail of safety in exploring an upper mediastinal hematoma.

▶   Never plunge blindly into the mediastinum in blunt trauma.

▶   Use Dacron for thoracic outlet arterial reconstructions.

▶   The phrenic nerve is your key to the subclavian artery.

▶   Go through the bed of the clavicle if the patient is bleeding.

Chapter 14
The Neck: Safari in Tiger Country

Go to the heart of danger, for there you will find safety.

~ Old Chinese proverb

The wounded neck is the anatomical "tiger country," a group of vital midline structures tightly packed together, carrying a large neurovascular bundle on each side. This delicate anatomy is just sitting inside a large hematoma waiting for you to make a wrong move. Even surgeons with elective experience in the neck will be challenged by a rapidly expanding cervical hematoma that obscures key landmarks and distorts the anatomy. To avoid getting lost in the injured neck, use the *trail of safety*, a well-defined sequence of steps that carefully guides you from one key anatomical landmark to the next without getting lost or causing iatrogenic damage.

TRAIL OF SAFETY

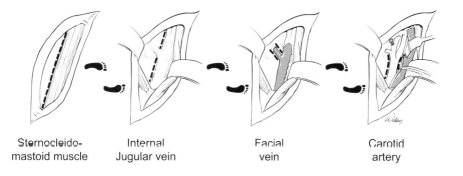

| Sternocleido-mastoid muscle | Internal Jugular vein | Facial vein | Carotid artery |

Follow a trail of safety in neck exploration

Before you begin

Always position the patient yourself. Improper positioning can turn a straightforward neck exploration into the safari from hell. Support the shoulders on a shoulder roll, and use a head support to extend and fully rotate the head to the other side. The superior mediastinum is an extension of the neck (Chapter 13), so your operative field extends from the mastoid process to the upper abdomen and includes both neck and chest. Never begin a neck exploration without a full set of vascular instruments, and remember to prepare a site for possible vein harvesting from the leg.

Making the incision

The utility incision for neck exploration runs along the anterior border of the sternocleidomastoid muscle (SCM). You can extend it from the mastoid process to the sternal notch, but a more limited incision is usually good enough. If you must go all the way to the sternal notch, you may be dealing with a thoracic outlet injury where proximal control must be gained in the chest. As you approach the angle of the mandible, curve your incision posteriorly to avoid the marginal mandibular branch of the facial nerve.

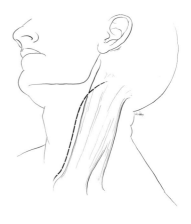

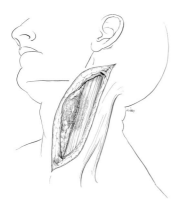

The first layer you encounter beneath the skin is the platysma. As it is divided, the edges of the incision open, and you are looking for the anterior border of the SCM, your first landmark on the trail of safety. This may not be easy in an injured neck with an expanding hematoma.

The most common pitfall is making your incision too posterior. If, upon dividing the platysma, you bump into longitudinal muscle fibers, move your dissection anteriorly. Gaining the anterior border of the SCM is more important than gaining the midline in a laparotomy incision. As you apply deliberate traction while your assistant applies countertraction, the incision almost opens itself.

> ### Gain the anterior border of the sternocleidomastoid

Develop your work space

Free the anterior border of the SCM by pulling it toward you and insert a self-retaining retractor below the muscle to keep the wound open. This is the first step in developing your work space.

You are now dissecting in the middle cervical fascia, the layer of areolar tissue beneath the retracted SCM. Your aim is to identify the internal jugular vein (IJ), your next landmark on the trail of safety.

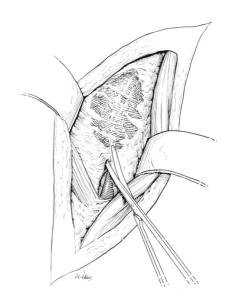

The IJ is the most commonly injured vascular structure in the neck. Temporarily control bleeding from this vessel with your finger or a small side-biting vascular clamp, and repair it using a 5:0 polypropylene suture. Don't hesitate to ligate the vein if repair is not straightforward. If the IJ is not injured, stay focused on its anterior border, which leads to the next landmark on the trail of safety - the facial vein.

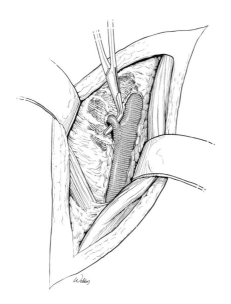

The facial vein is the gatekeeper of the neck, the key landmark you must identify, clamp, and ligate to open the way to the carotid bifurcation. Ligating and dividing it also allows you to continue developing your work space by repositioning the self-retaining retractor in a deeper layer so it pushes the IJ out of your way. You are now directly on top of the carotid artery. In most patients the facial vein is also a convenient marker for the level of the carotid bifurcation.

In the presence of a large hematoma, taking the necessary time to dissect out the facial vein is a smart move, even if you are in a hurry. Keep in mind that some patients have 2-3 small veins instead of one large facial vein, and all must be identified and divided along the anterior border of the IJ. A classic pitfall is mistaking the IJ for the facial vein and ligating it, only to make the dissection more difficult. You have negotiated the *trail of safety* through the injured neck. It's time to begin the next part of your operation: identifying and fixing the injuries.

The facial vein is the gatekeeper of the neck

The injured carotid

Gaining control

The cardinal principle of obtaining proximal control before entering a hematoma applies to carotid artery injury and means isolating the vessel in virgin territory proximal to the hematoma. You may occasionally have to

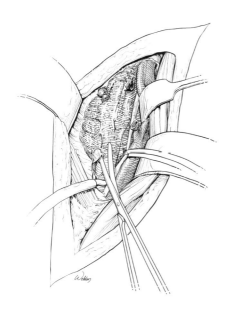

extend your incision to the sternal notch or even into a median sternotomy to obtain safe proximal control. Once inside the carotid sheath, find, identify, and protect the vagus nerve. Encircle the common carotid artery with a Rummel tourniquet and proceed with dissection toward the area of injury.

How about distal control? This is often problematic because a cervical hematoma typically extends up to the angle of the mandible (Chapter 3). Therefore, gaining distal control outside the hematoma may not be possible. Instead, prepare to gain distal control from *within* the hematoma. If you are ready for it, you can control back bleeding from the internal and external carotid arteries with minimal loss of blood.

As with any other named artery in the body, the safe plane along the carotid that protects you from mischief is the periadventitial plane (Chapter 3). As you reach the injury, you encounter back bleeding from the internal and external carotid arteries. First, use your finger for temporary control. Then, either clamp the distal artery or insert an intraluminal Fogarty catheter connected to a 3-way stopcock into the outflow tract. Remember that the hypoglossal nerve crosses over the proximal internal carotid, and the vagus nerve lies just behind it. You have come to the heart of tiger country, so stay in the safe periadventitial plane and bluntly push aside (rather than cut) any unidentified structures. Definitive control of the carotid bifurcation means occluding all three vessels: the common, internal, and external carotid arteries.

Once you have control of the injured carotid, talk to the anesthesiology team to assure the patient has a good blood pressure (a mean of at least 100mmHg) while the carotid is clamped. This is even more critical if backflow from the internal carotid is not very brisk.

Stay in the periadventitial plane of the carotid

Carotid repairs simplified

The carotid artery of a young healthy adult is surprisingly soft and pliable and doesn't tolerate abuse. Unless you are very gentle, you will end up with a torn artery or a repair that looks like a dog's breakfast and has to be redone.

There are many cool tricks for repairing the carotid artery, including such sophisticated maneuvers as transposition of the mobilized external carotid to connect it to the distal internal carotid. We advise you to keep it very simple and forget the cool stuff - or your patient will pay the price with a stroke. Use the simplest and fastest means to revascularize the brain.

Are there damage control options for a carotid injury? Definitely! We have no personal experience with temporary shunts in the carotid, but it makes perfect sense. If the patient is about to breach the physiological envelope or there are other more life-threatening injuries, ligation is a valid option. When considering ligation, remember the difference between the common and internal carotid arteries. Ligating the former is often well tolerated because the internal carotid remains perfused by backflow from the external carotid. Ligating the internal carotid, especially in a hypotensive patient, carries a significant risk of stroke. You may decide to take that risk to save the patient's life. Ligation is your only realistic option for inaccessible internal carotid injuries in Zone III. Some surgeons ligate the internal carotid artery if the patient has a profound neurological deficit (coma), while others reconstruct it regardless of the patient's neurological status. The prognosis is going to be very poor in either case.

What are the definitive repair options? On rare occasions, a clean laceration (usually a stab wound) may be amenable to simple lateral repair or end-to-end anastomosis. In most cases we use a synthetic graft or patch to reconstruct the carotid. We rarely use vein because it takes more time to harvest and prepare, and there is no good evidence that this makes the slightest difference.

Begin by exploring the injury. Open the artery longitudinally in the injured area to define the full extent of the damage. Carefully debride the contused or injured segment to obtain healthy arterial wall with a normal intima on all sides of the arterial defect. As you define the injury, plan ahead.

Precisely define the carotid injury

Your next step is thrombectomy to clear the inflow and outflow tracts. Carefully pass a No. 3 Fogarty balloon catheter proximally and distally. Don't push the catheter distally more than 2-3cm past the bifurcation - driving it through the carotid siphon will have spectacular results. Flush the proximal and distal ends of the injured artery with heparinized saline and begin the repair. If inserting an interposition graft, do the distal anastomosis first, especially if you are hooking up to the internal carotid above the bifurcation. It is difficult to work on the posterior wall of the distal anastomosis when the proximal anastomosis is already sewn in.

What should you do if there is no backflow from the distal internal carotid artery? This is a controversial point. We prefer to ligate the artery, for fear of converting an ischemic stroke into a hemorrhagic one. Some surgeons reconstruct the artery regardless of backflow.

If you have experience with elective carotid surgery and know how to smoothly insert a shunt and work around it - consider doing just that. A shunt is a smart move, especially if backflow from the internal carotid is weak or reconstruction is going to take time. Thread your shunt through the lumen of the interposition graft before insertion, and do the entire distal and most of the proximal anastomosis with the shunt in place.

A carotid injury in Zone III is uncommon and should ideally be identified preoperatively when your control options are either a Foley balloon catheter inserted into the missile tract or angiographic occlusion.

But what if you encounter a high internal carotid injury during an urgent exploration? You cannot reach the distal internal carotid without optimizing your exposure. In the presence of relentless back bleeding, you have no time for elaborate maneuvers such as subluxation of the jaw. Your best bet is a much simpler alternative - a muscular and determined assistant armed with a suitable retractor. Extend your incision to the mastoid process, insert a retractor into the upper corner of the wound, and have your assistant pull really hard, giving you a few critical millimeters. If this is not enough, divide the posterior belly of the digastric muscle to gain more room.

When all you can see is the bleeding orifice of the internal carotid, ligation of the artery is your only realistic option. The injury is simply too high for reconstruction. If there isn't even enough length to ligate or apply a metal clip, consider inserting a Fogarty catheter into the bleeding orifice and inflating it. Apply two metal clips across the catheter very close to the balloon, and cut the catheter proximally, leaving the permanently inflated balloon inside the artery. It may not be the most elegant solution in the book - but it works.

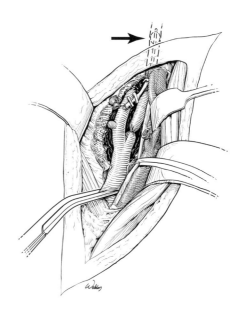

Ligating the carotid is not a crime

Exsanguination from bone

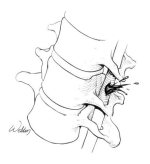

Have you ever seen exsanguinating hemorrhage from a hole in a bone? This is how a vertebral artery injury often presents in the open neck. In the era of liberal angiography, this should be a rare situation because the preferred management of vertebral artery injuries is angiographic, not operative. Occasionally, however, you will discover that the carotid sheath is intact while audible arterial bleeding is spurting from a hole in the paravertebral muscles lateral and posterior to it. Feel for the bodies of the cervical vertebrae to orient yourself, and you will realize that bleeding is coming from the area of the transverse processes. If you swipe the paravertebral muscles laterally with a periosteal elevator, you are met with the unforgettable sight of brisk hemorrhage from a hole in a bone, the bone being the transverse process of the injured cervical vertebra.

The several ingenious techniques described for this exotic injury are a sure sign that many creative surgeons have found it a baffling problem. Unroofing the injured artery in its bony canal is a demanding technical feat even under the best elective circumstances. We certainly don't consider it a feasible option in a bleeding patient, and neither should you. Proximal control of the injured artery at the base of the neck will not control backflow from the brain.

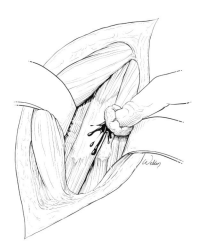

Here, again, the simplest solution is the best. Pushing a piece of bone wax into the bleeding hole usually works like magic! If your facility has angiographic capabilities, immediate postoperative angiogram with embolization of the injured vertebral artery is another option.

> **Use bone wax to plug a hosing vertebral artery**

The esophagus

There are two routes to the cervical esophagus, going either medial or lateral to the carotid sheath. The medial route is a natural continuation of carotid exploration and probably the one which you are most familiar with.

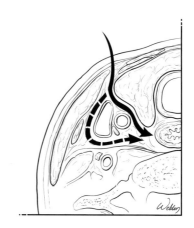

Before exploring the esophagus, ask the anesthesiologist to insert a large-bore nasogastric tube to help you identify the esophagus by palpating the tube in a hostile operative field. The esophagus is located slightly to the left of the midline, making it easier to explore from the left side of the neck.

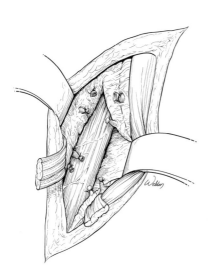

Retract the content of the carotid sheath laterally and enter the plane between it and the trachea. You will find the esophagus behind the trachea and anterior to the spine. Full exposure of the esophagus requires you identify and divide three structures that cross over the esophagus: the omohyoid muscle, middle thyroid vein, and inferior thyroid artery. The recurrent laryngeal nerve is rarely identified in the injured hostile neck.

The other approach to the esophagus, going lateral to the carotid artery, is a "back door" approach, useful when a large hematoma in the carotid sheath obscures the anatomy. Retract the carotid sheath structures medially instead of laterally, and enter the plane between the carotid sheath and the cervical spine to find the esophagus. Your work space is limited, but you are less likely to cause iatrogenic damage.

Approach the injured esophagus through a front or back door

Esophageal injuries are not easy to identify because the esophagus doesn't have serosa. If you can't be sure there is an injury, guide the anesthesiologist to pull the nasogastric tube to the level of your exploration, flood the operative field with saline, and ask the anesthesiologist to inflate the nasogastric tube with air. Watch for emerging air bubbles.

The most worrisome aspect of an esophageal exploration is not what you can see and feel, but what you *can't*. Is there an injury to the other side of the esophagus? To the posterior wall? With limited exposure, it is easy to miss such an injury. If you suspect a hole you can't see, here are your options:

◆ Contralateral neck exploration through a separate incision - often your safest choice.
◆ Intraoperative esophagoscopy to look for an injury from inside the lumen.
◆ Mobilize the esophagus by bluntly developing the plane between it, the trachea anteriorly, and the anterior longitudinal ligaments posteriorly. Hook your finger (or a Penrose drain) around it and inspect the contralateral and posterior aspects. However, this maneuver is more difficult than our description leads you to believe, especially if you are trying to do it through a right-sided neck incision. Unless you have decent experience with esophageal surgery, don't use this option. You may cause iatrogenic injury to the esophagus and recurrent laryngeal nerves, as well as devascularize the trachea.

Regardless of the option you choose, the key tactical principle is to be sure about the hidden aspects of the esophagus before concluding your exploration.

Worry about the hidden aspects of the esophagus

After identifying an esophageal injury, carefully assess the extent of damage. Mucosal damage is often more extensive than the apparent injury to the muscularis. Conservatively debride the wound to obtain healthy edges on all sides and repair it using one or two layers. Our preference is a single layer repair using an absorbable monofilament suture. Much more important than the number of layers is precise definition and meticulous approximation of the mucosal defect without tension.

Always isolate your esophageal repair from other suture lines. If you have also fixed the carotid artery or the trachea, remember that the esophageal repair is the one most likely to fail. When it fails - it may take your other repairs with it. Don't let it happen. Interpose a well-vascularized chunk of healthy muscle between the esophagus and any adjacent suture lines. The strap muscles, omohyoid or sternal head of the SCM can each be transected close to their inferior attachments and then used to keep your suture lines safely apart.

What is the damage control option for the cervical esophagus? Since the aim is to prevent an uncontrolled leak, the bail out solution is external drainage. If the injury is inaccessible (e.g. high or posterior in the hypopharynx), just drain it. If there is no distal obstruction, the fistula will rapidly close.

When you cannot safely close the defect because it is too large, the operation was delayed, or you have to bail out, either drain or exteriorize it as a lateral esophagostomy. This is particularly relevant when you encounter combined injuries to the esophagus and trachea, where creating two high-risk suture lines is asking for trouble. Repairing the airway and diverting the esophagus may be a safer option.

A quick and easy bail out option that has worked for us is to insert a large suction drain into the defect, rapidly purse-string the esophageal wall around it and bring it out through the skin. Whatever you choose as your damage control solution, remember: an uncontrolled esophageal leak means mediastinitis and death; a controlled fistula means a longer hospital stay with a good chance of recovery.

Bail out by creating a controlled esophageal fistula

The larynx and trachea

Injuries to the upper airway come in two types: small and large. Repair small lacerations of the larynx and trachea with interrupted 3:0 monofilament absorbable sutures tied on the outside. Never use non-absorbable sutures to repair the airway.

Large defects cannot be simply approximated without tension because part of the cartilage is missing. To obtain a good outcome, you are well advised to get early help from an ENT colleague. They have more experience with the upper airway and will ultimately manage any complications.

Several damage control options for upper airway injuries are available. You can simply push the endotracheal tube past the injured area to eliminate the air leak, leaving the injury alone for a delayed reconstruction. Another option is tracheostomy. Inserting a tracheostomy tube through a traumatic tracheal defect is not a good move under elective circumstances. It is, however, perfectly acceptable as a bail out option when the patient has other life-threatening injuries, or when you are facing a complex injury on your own.

Transcervical injuries

How should you approach a penetrating injury that crosses the neck from side-to-side? Transcervical injuries may require bilateral exploration. Ruling out an injury to the other side of the esophagus or trachea by intraoperative endoscopy, while technically possible, is logistically cumbersome.

To explore a transcervical penetration, we prefer a U incision, the cervical equivalent of a clam-shell thoracotomy. If you spend a few minutes developing a superior skin flap in the subplatysma plane (as you would do in a thyroidectomy), you gain maximal exposure of the bilateral neck, much like lifting the hood of your car to look at the engine. Exposure just doesn't get any better than this.

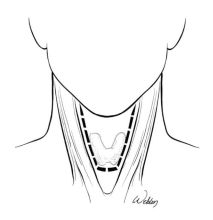

Lift the hood off the neck with a U incision

Finishing up

Have a good look at the edges of your incision in search of superficial bleeders. In the neck, a small muscular bleeder can easily lead to a postoperative expanding hematoma and the need for urgent re-exploration. Inspect your suture lines and make sure they are nicely separated by viable muscle.

We strongly advise you drain every neck exploration for trauma using a closed suction drain. The most commonly missed injury in the neck is a small esophageal perforation. Your drain will convert a potential disaster into a minor problem. If draining an esophageal suture line, bring your drain out anteriorly without crossing over the carotid artery - drains have been known to erode into it. The only layer you have to approximate deep to the skin is the platysma. Then close the skin and you have successfully completed your safari in tiger country.

THE KEY POINTS

▶   Follow a trail of safety in neck exploration.

▶   Gain the anterior border of the sternocleidomastoid.

▶   The facial vein is the gatekeeper of the neck.

▶   Stay in the periadventitial plane of the carotid.

▶   Precisely define the carotid injury.

▶   Ligating the carotid is not a crime.

▶   Use bone wax to plug a hosing vertebral artery.

▶   Approach the injured esophagus through a front or back door.

▶   Worry about the hidden aspects of the esophagus.

▶   Bail out by creating a controlled esophageal fistula.

▶   Lift the hood off the neck with a U incision.

Chapter 15

Peripheral Vascular Trauma Made Simple

Everything should be made as simple as possible, but not simpler.

~ Albert Einstein

If you think you know what a bloody mess looks like, a close encounter with a hosing groin will have you think again. The patient is in shock, with most of the blood volume either left at the scene or all over the paramedic compressing the bleeding groin for dear life. Since this is one of the most spectacular penetrating injuries, it is easy to forget priorities, make critical errors, and lose the patient in the midst of the chaos.

In this chapter we try to bridge the wide gap between the neat illustrations of vascular exposures you see in books and the harsh reality of the OR, where the patient is bleeding and all you can see in the operative field is traumatized muscle and lots of hematoma. Bridging this gap is especially important for surgeons who don't do peripheral vascular work on a regular basis but are called upon to control and repair the occasional arterial injury. Our key message is that the injured artery is always part of a wounded patient, and the patient's overall trauma burden often dictates how you approach the vascular injury.

Gaining control of the hosing groin

Obtain temporary control of the bleeding groin with local pressure applied by an enthusiastic assistant or a Foley catheter in the tract. Once in the OR, you need proximal control and have three options:

◆ Laparotomy - if there is urgent indication, go into the abdomen and control the external iliac artery in the pelvis.

◆ Retroperitoneal approach - expose the external iliac artery through an oblique lower abdominal incision approximately 2cm above and parallel to the inguinal ligament. Incise the aponeuroses of the external and internal oblique, and open the transversus abdominis and transversalis fascia to expose the preperitoneal fat. Gentle cephalad retraction of the peritoneal sac will bring you to the external iliac artery. This approach avoids laparotomy, but takes time, so is rarely used in the bleeding patient.

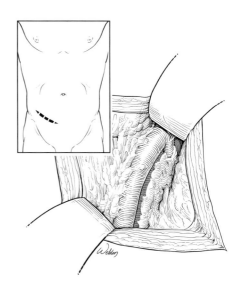

◆ Vertical groin incision - the simplest way to gain proximal control of the hosing groin.

So much for the good news. The bad news is that even with proximal control, the patient continues to bleed, albeit at a slower rate. If back bleeding is not very brisk and you can identify the key structures, use a combination of sharp and blunt dissection to expose the femoral vessels. Blunt dissection is safer in hostile territory. You want to avoid damage to the femoral nerve, and you cannot cut the femoral nerve with your finger.

If you can't see what you're doing because of brisk back bleeding, walk the clamps (Chapter 9). The source of persistent back bleeding is often the deep femoral artery that must be identified and controlled. When you succeed, breath a sigh of relief; you have successfully dealt with one of the cobras of trauma surgery.

Gain proximal control of the hosing groin

A quick tour of the femoral triangle

You are probably familiar with the femoral triangle from visits to the groin in elective vascular procedures. Make a vertical skin incision over the femoral pulse, if present. Otherwise, place your incision halfway between the pubic tubercle and the anterior superior iliac spine. Approximately one-third of the incision should extend above the groin crease. This is not the time to be hesitant or minimally invasive.

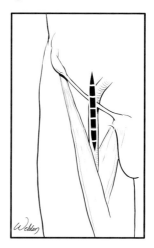

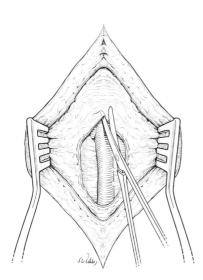

Exposing the femoral vessels in a war zone is not easy. You have to identify and incise two fascial layers: the fascia lata and the femoral sheath. Cut the fascia lata longitudinally to enter the fat of the femoral triangle and insert a self-retaining retractor. Your best friend in the hostile groin is the inguinal ligament, and the experienced surgeon makes a point of identifying it early. Palpate the fatty content of the triangle with an educated finger. Feel for a pulse or, if absent, for a tubular structure in the fat. In the pulseless groin, you often encounter muscle beneath the fascia lata. This simply means that you are too lateral, over the iliopsoas muscle, so redirect your dissection medially.

The inguinal ligament is your only friend in a hostile groin

Next, open the femoral sheath to identify the femoral artery. Reposition the self-retaining retractor at a deeper level or add another retractor. Stay on top of the artery in the periadventitial plane. If you deviate medially, you may be greeted by a gush of dark blood from the femoral vein. If you stray laterally, you may injure the femoral nerve.

Isolate and control the common femoral artery and its branches. While the common and superficial femoral arteries can be readily identified and encircled in the proximal and distal parts of the incision, isolating the deep femoral artery can be difficult for surgeons with few "groin hours." The lateral femoral circumflex vein is the most treacherous vein in the groin. It crosses immediately in front

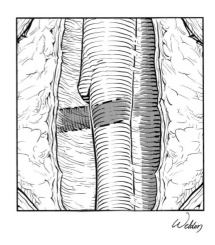

of the proximal deep femoral artery in the crotch between the deep and superficial femoral artery. If you try to expose the deep femoral artery by unroofing it, you soon encounter brisk venous bleeding from the injured vein. Avoiding this unpleasant situation is far better than trying to fix it. Do not dissect out the deep femoral artery, plain and simple!

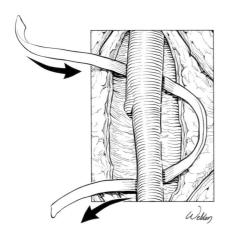

The origin of the deep femoral artery is marked by an abrupt change in the diameter of the common femoral artery. Take a vessel loop and pass one end from lateral to medial underneath the common femoral artery well above the bifurcation. Grab the other end of the loop and pass it from medial to lateral well below the bifurcation. Lift up both ends of the loop to discover that you have neatly isolated the deep femoral artery without dissecting it out.

Don't dissect out the deep femoral artery

Getting around the groin is more difficult in the presence of a sizeable hematoma. We call it a hostile groin, and when you come face-to-face with it, you will see why. The anatomy is distorted, the tissues are suffused with blood, and a bulging hematoma is looking up at you in total defiance.

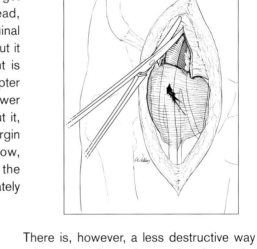

Here, we would like to let you in on a little trade secret. Forget the femoral vessels! Instead, focus on finding the inguinal ligament. It sounds crazy - but it works. The inguinal ligament is an anatomical barrier (Chapter 3), and if you identify the lower edge of the ligament and cut it, you will find yourself in the virgin lower retroperitoneum. Now, you can easily identify the external iliac vessels immediately above the groin.

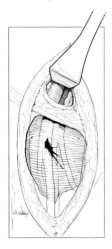

There is, however, a less destructive way to clamp the femoral vessels above the inguinal ligament. Take blunt Mayo scissors and make a hole in the inguinal ligament approximately 1-2cm above and parallel to its edge. Insert a narrow deep retractor to keep the space open. This brings you into the hematoma-free retroperitoneum without dividing the inguinal ligament. You can now use this hole to easily palpate and safely clamp the external iliac artery above the groin. All this is very cool, but if you are pressed for time and the groin is actively bleeding, don't hesitate to cut the inguinal ligament. It is a small price to pay for expedient proximal control.

Control the common femoral artery through the inguinal ligament

---

Considering your options

As in any other operation for trauma, you now have to choose an operative profile. Consider the patient's overall trauma burden and physiology, as well as the operative circumstances (Chapter 1). Are you operating in a university trauma center or in an improvised field hospital in a war zone? How comfortable are you with vascular work? Balance all these against the repair options.

Damage control options for the femoral vessels are temporary shunting or ligation. A temporary shunt in the common or superficial femoral artery is an excellent damage control solution to maintain distal perfusion. We strongly recommend you do a pre-emptive fasciotomy to give the leg added protection in case of early shunt failure (Chapter 3). On very rare occasions when a shunt is not an option, ligating the femoral artery is a valid alternative. In fact, you can ligate the superficial femoral artery in a young healthy patient with low risk of limb loss, provided collateral circulation via the deep femoral artery is intact. In the great majority of bail out situations, a shunt is a much better option.

When operating in damage control mode, fix the femoral vein only if you can get away with a simple lateral repair. Don't hesitate to ligate the vein if the injury requires anything more elaborate.

Shunt + fasciotomy = bail out for femoral artery injuries

Preserving the deep femoral artery, when possible, is an important principle. Your ability to reconstruct the bifurcation depends on your vascular experience and technical repertoire. One well-known trick in the face of extensive damage to the bifurcation is to join the stumps of the superficial and deep femoral arteries side-to-side to create a short common arterial trunk before inserting an interposition graft. This spares you the awkward job of implanting the deep femoral artery into the graft.

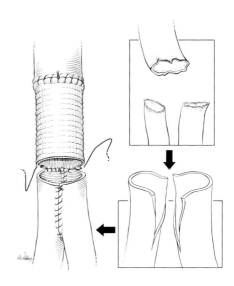

If the posterior wall of the injured femoral artery is intact, do a patch repair. If the artery is transected, interpose a synthetic graft or a reversed saphenous vein from the other leg. If the arterial and venous suture lines are immediately adjacent, interpose viable muscle between them to prevent an arteriovenous fistula. We do not insert interposition grafts into the femoral vein, but many surgeons do.

Whatever you do to fix the femoral vessels, plan your reconstruction with soft tissue coverage in mind. If you cannot cover the arterial reconstruction with well-vascularized soft tissue (e.g. swinging the sartorius muscle over the repair), call someone who can. An exposed arterial suture line is a ticking time bomb that will blow up in your face.

An exposed vascular suture line is a ticking time bomb

The superficial femoral artery

Not surprisingly, a description of superficial femoral artery exposures is not found in most vascular surgical atlases because it is rarely used in elective surgery. Here's how it's done.

Slightly flex and externally rotate the patient's leg, supporting it on folded towels. When working above the knee, support the

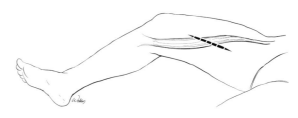

leg below the knee to avoid distorting your work space. Make a longitudinal incision over the anterior border of the sartorius muscle, extending it well proximal to the injury. Incise the skin carefully to avoid accidentally transecting

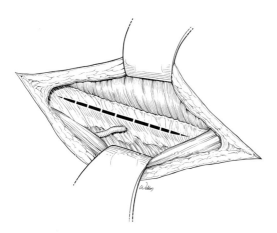

the saphenous vein. Open the superficial fascia and identify the sartorius muscle, the gatekeeper of the superficial femoral artery. Retract the sartorius, either anteriorly (in the upper and middle thigh) or posteriorly (in the middle and lower thigh), by inserting a self-retaining retractor into the wound. Your target is the fibrous roof of Hunter's canal, the

white fascia directly underneath the sartorius between the adductor magnus and vastus medialis muscles. Open it and you are staring at the neurovascular bundle. Carefully free the superficial femoral artery from the

adjacent vein and pay special attention to the saphenous nerve that is part of the neurovascular bundle and can be easily damaged. As with any vascular injury, start your dissection in virgin territory proximal to the injury, and proceed distally toward the injured segment.

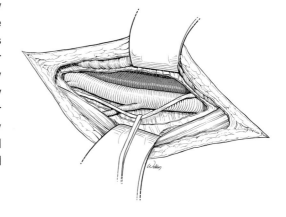

What are your repair options? You may elect to insert a shunt if you need to bail out or if you decide (with the orthopedic surgeons) to achieve bone alignment prior to arterial repair. This is generally a good idea since sewing a graft in an unstable flailing limb is something you should avoid if possible. When the superficial femoral artery is transected, insert an interposition graft.

The sartorius is the gatekeeper of the superficial femoral artery

---

Popliteal repairs the easy way

Treat the popliteal artery with the respect it deserves. It is the least accessible vessel in the lower extremity, and the collateral flow around the knee is insufficient to sustain viability of the lower leg if flow in the popliteal artery is interrupted. Even today, popliteal artery trauma carries the highest limb loss rate of all extremity vascular injuries.

Always begin a popliteal repair with fasciotomy, even if you are an extremely smooth operator. If there are no associated injuries that may bleed, give systemic heparin. Many popliteal repairs fail because of clotted distal microcirculation, not because of a technical flaw.

Treat the injured popliteal artery with the greatest respect

The safe and sound route to the injured popliteal artery is the medial approach. Make an incision in the lower thigh along the palpable groove between the vastus medialis and sartorius muscles. Palpate 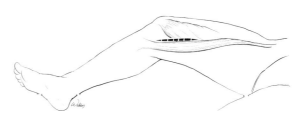 the posterior border of the femur and incise the deep fascia posterior to it, bringing you straight into the fatty content of the popliteal fossa. Insert a finger and palpate the pulse of the popliteal artery against the posterior aspect of

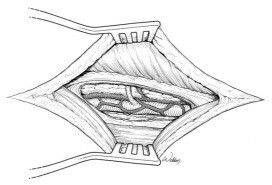

the femur. The posterior edge of the bone is the key anatomical landmark to identify the popliteal vessels, both above and below the knee. Now identify, dissect out, and encircle the above-knee popliteal artery. The three major pitfalls in this dissection are injuring the closely adherent popliteal vein, cutting the saphenous nerve, and mistaking the vein for the artery.

Find the popliteal artery immediately behind the bone

Expose the distal popliteal segment through a separate incision that runs approximately 1cm behind the border of the tibia, beginning at the level of the knee immediately posterior to the medial femoral condyle.

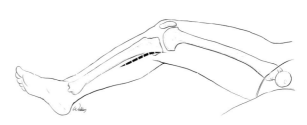

Again, beware of injuring the saphenous vein that lies immediately posterior to your incision. Cutting the deep fascia reveals the fat of the distal popliteal fossa, where you find the neurovascular bundle immediately behind the bone. The first structure

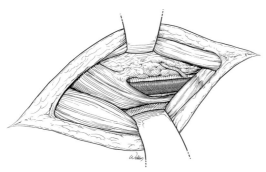

you encounter is the popliteal vein, and you have to carefully dissect the artery away from it.

So much for proximal and distal control. But how are you going to fix the injury itself, an injury that still remains hidden behind the knee? Well, you can do it the hard way or the easy way.

The hard way is the traditional full popliteal exposure, the one you should describe in your Board Exam because this is what examiners expect to hear. It entails joining the medial incisions above and below the knee and dividing the tendinous attachments of the posteromedial muscles (sartorius, gracilis, semimembranosus, semitendinosus), as well as the attachment of the medial head of the gastrocnemius. In practice, grab the cautery and blaze a trail of destruction between your proximal and distal incisions, blasting any tendon that stands between you and the popliteal artery. It sounds like a search and destroy mission because it is. By the time you finish, it is not a pretty sight, but you can get to the artery and fix it.

There is a simpler alternative. Instead of exposing the injured artery, bypass and exclude it. You already have the proximal and distal popliteal segments looped and ready. Even if the popliteal vein is injured, it doesn't matter. You don't have to reconstruct it to achieve a good outcome. The notion that you do is just another sacred cow that has been slaughtered by current data. Your most expedient solution is to harvest a piece of saphenous vein from the other thigh, reverse it, and insert it as an interposition graft between the proximal and distal popliteal artery, excluding the injured segment.

Bluntly create an inter-condylar tunnel between the proximal and distal incisions. Do a longitudinal arteriotomy in the proximal popliteal artery above the knee, hook up the reversed vein end-to-side, and then doubly ligate the artery immediately distal

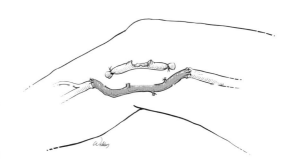

to the anastomosis to exclude the injured segment. Pass the pulsating graft through the tunnel, and hook it up to a similar arteriotomy in the distal popliteal artery below the knee. Then ligate the artery immediately proximal to the distal anastomosis to complete the exclusion. In an obese patient with a deep artery, it is easier to transect the proximal and distal popliteal artery, oversew the ends of the excluded segment, and then hook up the vein graft end-to-end.

The huge advantage of this approach is simplicity. You don't have to deal with the injured segment at all. The only valid reason to take down the ligaments and expose the popliteal fossa is ongoing bleeding from the injured segment despite exclusion, a situation we have yet to encounter.

> **Bypass and exclude the injured popliteal artery**

Below the knee

Reconstructing a tibial artery in a patient with a blunt "bumper" injury that includes a fractured tibia and fibula is an experience likely to remain etched in your memory. Imagine spending the better part of an on-call night trying to bridge two spastic noodles in a soup of blood, broken bones, and torn muscles. Answering the following three questions can help make this experience much less traumatic for you and your patient.

1. Is this escapade really necessary? One of the three leg arteries open all the way down to the foot is good enough. The traditional teaching that patients with blunt trauma need two open vessels is an unsubstantiated urban legend. Remember - if one of the three arteries is bleeding, the solution is not surgical exploration and ligation, but, rather, angiographic occlusion of the bleeder (unless angiography is not available).

2. Do you have the required information for a safe trip? Starting a vascular exploration below the knee without a clear angiographic delineation of the injured segment is like starting the Dakar Rally without a map. Make every effort to obtain a formal angiogram. If you

are forced to run to the OR urgently, begin by exposing the popliteal artery below the knee and shooting an on-table angiogram. A suboptimal angiogram can send you on a lengthy exploration of what turns out to be an intact artery in spasm.

3. Where to begin? The popliteal fossa below the knee is an excellent starting point because you can always find the artery there, even if you have little vascular experience. It is virgin territory, the vessels are large, and you can identify the neurovascular bundle and follow it distally.

Retract the medial head of the gastroc-nemius posteriorly and expose the edge of the soleus muscle arching over the popliteal vessels. Hook a finger underneath the muscle and detach it from the tibia. This opens the space, allowing you to place a self-retaining retractor in the wound. Proceed distally toward the injury by taking

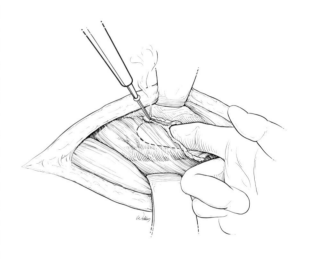

down the attachment of the soleus to the posterior aspect of the tibia. Look for the anterior tibial vein as a marker of the take-off of the anterior

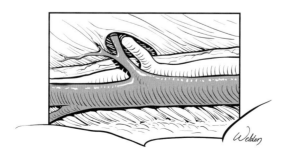

tibial artery. Further distally, identify the bifurcation of the tibioperoneal trunk into the posterior tibial and peroneal arteries, where the former is the more superficial vessel.

Expose the anterior tibial artery in the mid- and lower leg through your anterior fasciotomy incision. Insert a self-retaining retractor between the tibialis anterior and the extensor hallucis longus muscles, and find the neurovascular bundle deep down between the muscles, on the interosseus membrane.

Before you begin a vascular exploration below the knee, strongly consider using a proximal pneumatic tourniquet above the knee. Nothing is more frustrating than trying to identify and isolate the small and fragile vessels of the lower leg in the presence of active bleeding, not to mention the increased risk of iatrogenic injury to other elements of the neurovascular bundle.

Which artery should you reconstruct? Always go for the most straightforward solution in the most accessible artery and take into account soft tissue coverage. Most often, this translates into reconstructing the posterior tibial artery. In a badly injured leg, be prepared to spend some time looking for the distal end of the transected vessel, which may be difficult to find. In most instances, your best reconstructive option is an interposition graft using a reversed saphenous vein from the other ankle.

One open tibial artery is good enough

The axillary artery

To gain rapid access to the proximal axillary artery, you have to go through the pectoralis major muscle. Abduct the arm and make an infraclavicular incision extending from the mid-clavicle to the deltopectoral groove. This transpectoral route is an extensile exposure. You can extend it distally along the deltopectoral groove. Dissection between the deltoid and the pectoralis major, combined with

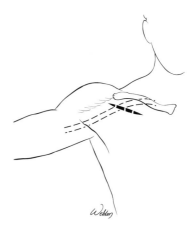

lateral retraction of the cephalic vein, will reveal the clavipectoral fascia containing the neurovascular bundle. Further distal extension into the groove between the biceps and the triceps muscles will get you to the proximal brachial artery.

Cut down to the pectoral fascia, divide it, and then spread the pectoralis major fibers by inserting closed Mayo scissors into the muscle and opening them perpendicular to the fibers to make a hole. Underneath you find the pectoralis minor and the clavipectoral fascia medial to it. Open the clavipectoral fascia and dissect in the axillary fat to identify the axillary vein, the gatekeeper of the axilla. The artery is deep and superior to it. To optimize your work space, get the pectoralis minor muscle out of the way either by retracting it laterally or dividing its upper attachment to the coracoid process. To safely mobilize the axillary artery, you must first identify, clamp, and cut the thoracoacromial artery, one of the only arterial branches in the body to come straight at you when exposing the parent vessel.

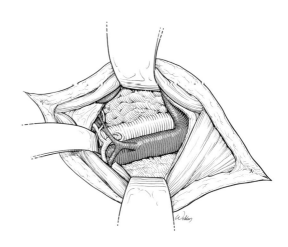

Your damage control options for axillary artery injuries are shunt insertion and, less commonly, ligation and fasciotomy. Ample collaterals around the shoulder will prevent critical distal ischemia in most patients with an interrupted axillary artery, but reconstruction (using a saphenous vein graft harvested from the thigh) is a better option if feasible.

Approach the axillary artery through the pectoralis major, not around it

The brachial artery

The brachial artery is the most frequently injured artery in the body and certainly one of the most accessible. Gain access to the proximal artery via a medial upper arm incision along the groove between the biceps and triceps muscles. This incision is the epitome of extensile exposure, as it can be easily extended both proximally into the deltopectoral groove and distally across the antecubital fossa into the forearm. Incise the deep fascia at the medial border of the biceps,

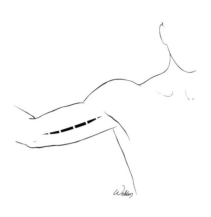

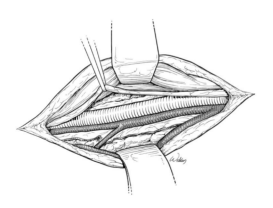

taking care to avoid iatrogenic injury to the basilic vein as it emerges through the fascia in the lower aspect of the incision. Anterior retraction of the biceps will expose the neurovascular bundle enveloped in the brachial sheath. The first structure you encounter (and your landmark) is the median nerve. Retract it gently to get it out of your way.

Distal extension of the medial arm incision is via an S-shaped incision carried across the antecubital space distal to the skin crease. The distal brachial artery and its bifurcation are located immediately beneath the biceps tendon, again in close proximity to the median nerve.

The damage control option for the brachial artery is ligation and fasciotomy, which is very well tolerated, especially if the injury is in the mid- or distal arm beyond to the take-off of the deep brachial artery. The definitive repair option is a vein interposition graft using the saphenous vein harvested above the ankle.

THE KEY POINTS

▶ Gain proximal control of the hosing groin.

▶ The inguinal ligament is your only friend in a hostile groin.

▶ Don't dissect out the deep femoral artery.

▶ Control the common femoral artery through the inguinal ligament.

▶ Shunt + fasciotomy = bail out for femoral artery injuries.

▶ An exposed vascular suture line is a ticking time bomb.

▶ The sartorius is the gatekeeper of the superficial femoral artery.

▶ Treat the injured popliteal artery with the greatest respect.

▶ Find the popliteal artery immediately behind the bone.

▶ Bypass and exclude the injured popliteal artery.

▶ One open tibial artery is good enough.

▶ Approach the axillary artery through the pectoralis major, not around it.

Epilogue
The Joy of Trauma Surgery

*This book has cost me much time and trouble.
I have written it slowly, and I might say that
I have lived it before writing it.*

~ Felix Lejars, *Urgent Surgery*,
Translated from the French 6th Edition
New York, Wood, 1910

This book is a genuine effort to come as close as possible to teaching trauma surgery *in vivo* using the principles, techniques, and tricks we share with our residents every day across the operating table. The single most important principle we teach is to *always keep it simple*, because in trauma surgery, the simple stuff works. Once out of training, you rapidly discover that complex techniques and sophisticated maneuvers make for neat illustrations - but often result in dead patients. The sicker your patient is, the simpler and quicker your operative solution must be.

Can you learn to operate from a book? Some experts claim this is as futile as trying to learn Kung Fu from a web site. We don't agree. Much of what we do and teach in the OR comes from the wisdom and experience of old masters we have never even met. Through the printed page, they have reached across generations and continents to guide our hand in times of trouble. Their wise advice, based on practical experience, has worked amazingly well for us. Although we are still around and not particularly hard to reach (asher.hirshberg@gmail.com and kmattox@bcm.tmc.edu), we hope the advice we offer in *Top Knife* will do the same for you.

We have found trauma surgery an immensely rewarding field, a perpetually fascinating challenge, and a source of professional pride and joy. Beyond the strategic thinking, tactical decisions, technical tricks and adrenaline rush, our overriding motivating force is always the critically injured patient. Regardless of your chosen field or specialty, we trust you will always be there for the severely wounded patients who put their lives in your hands.

Asher Hirshberg and Kenneth Mattox
August 2004